Constipation

Edited by Gyula Mózsik

Published in London, United Kingdom

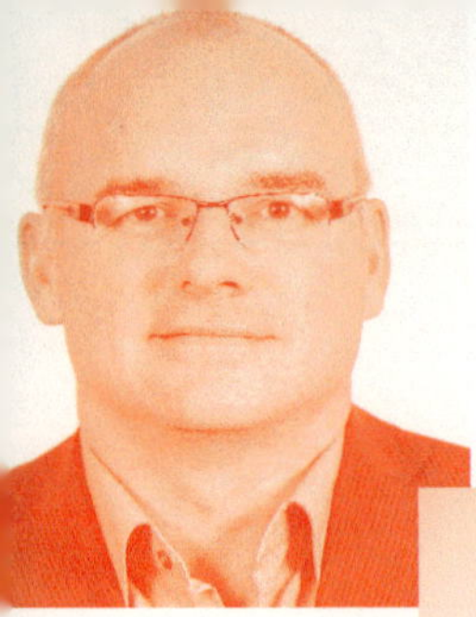
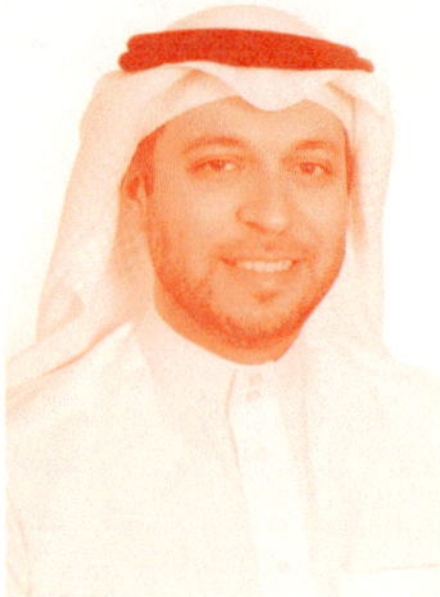
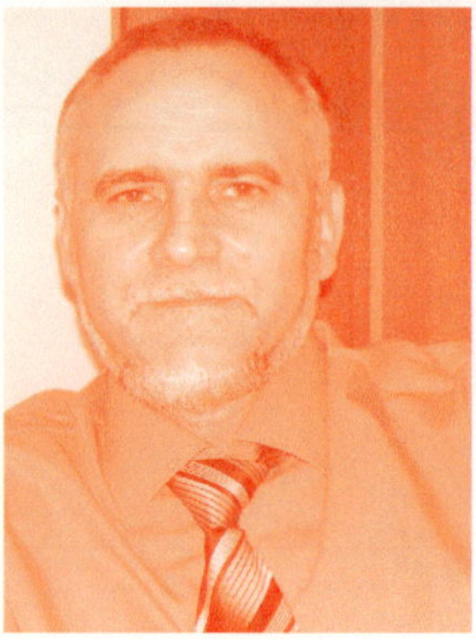
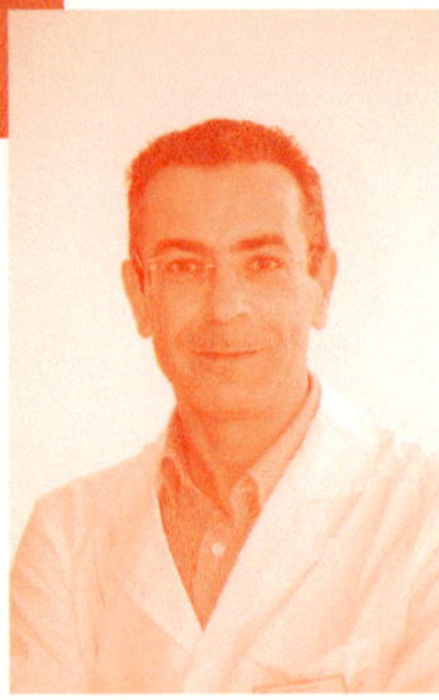
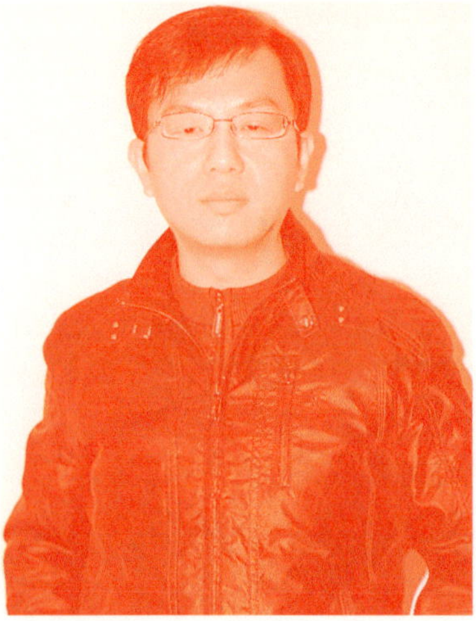
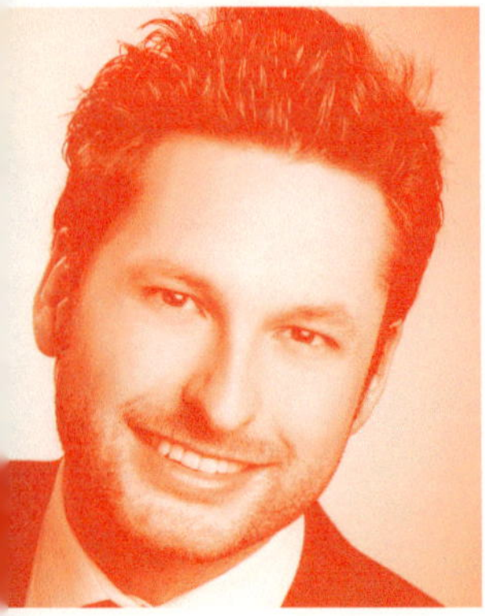
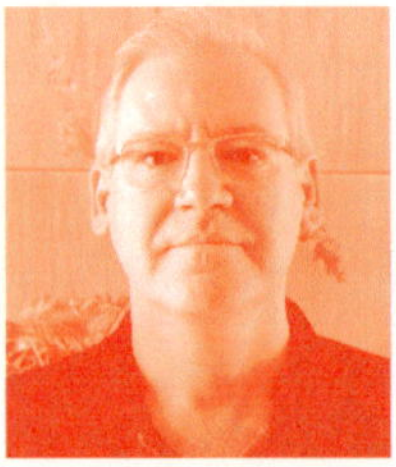

IntechOpen

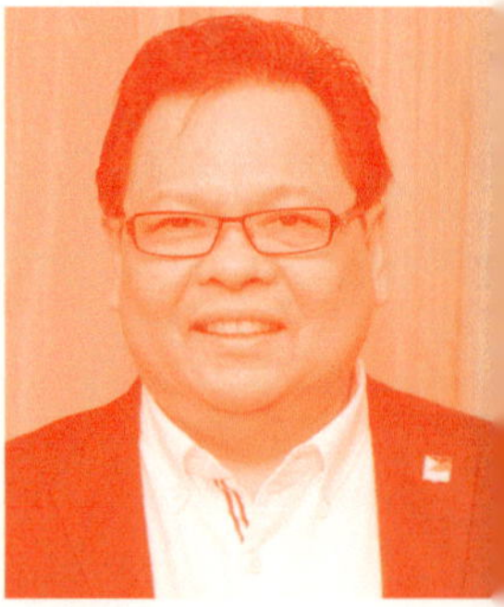
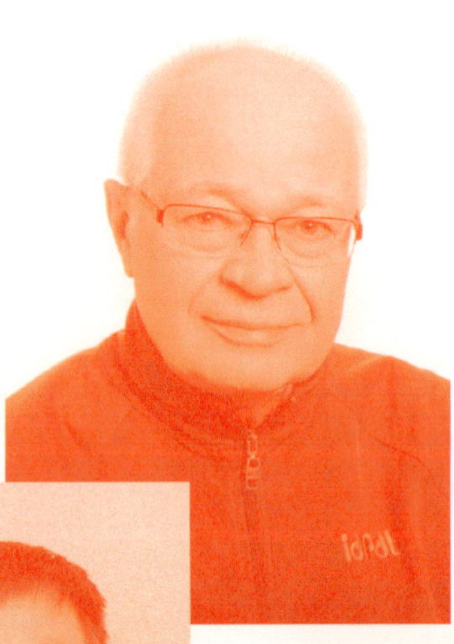
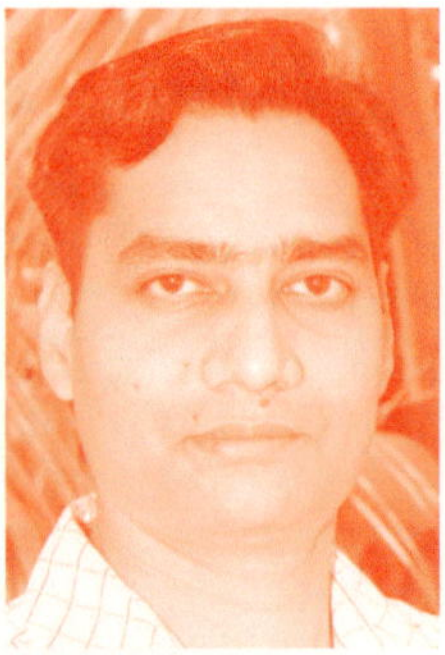
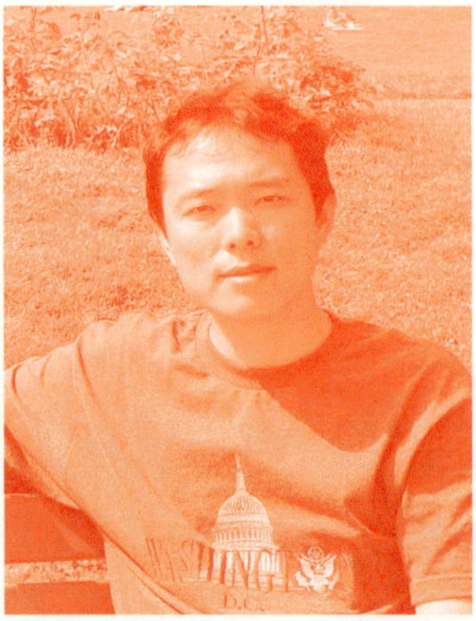
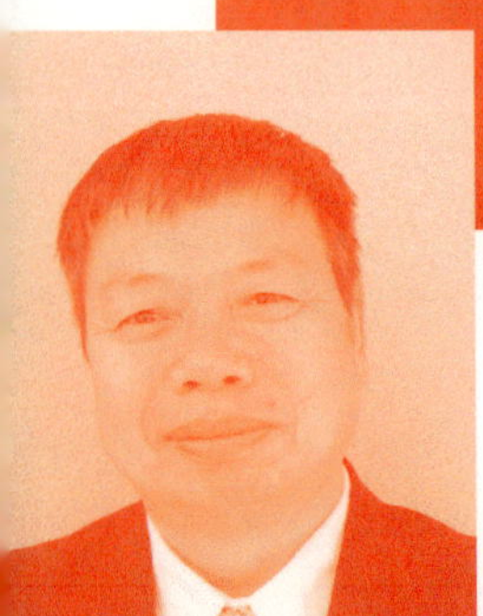
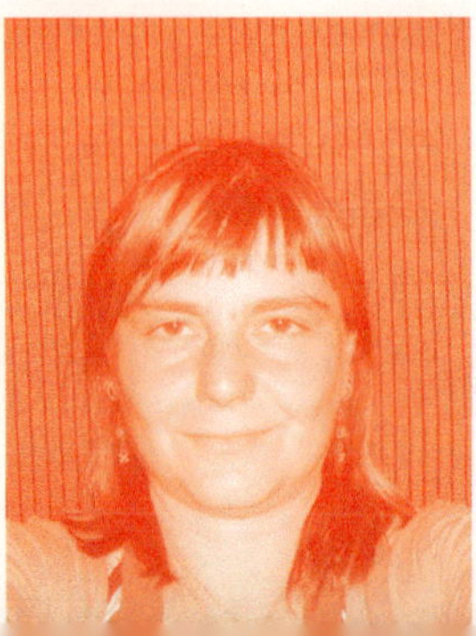

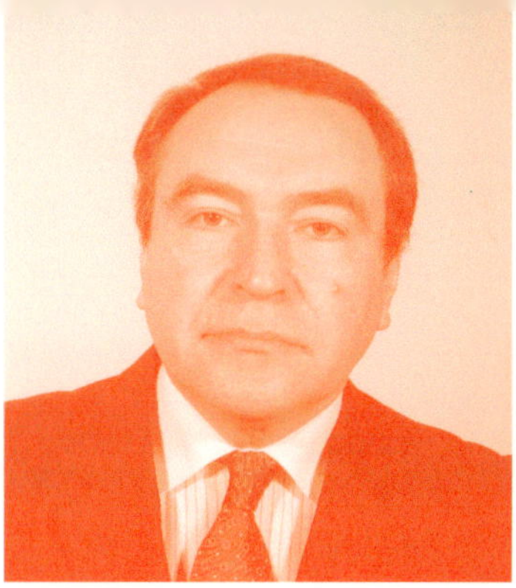
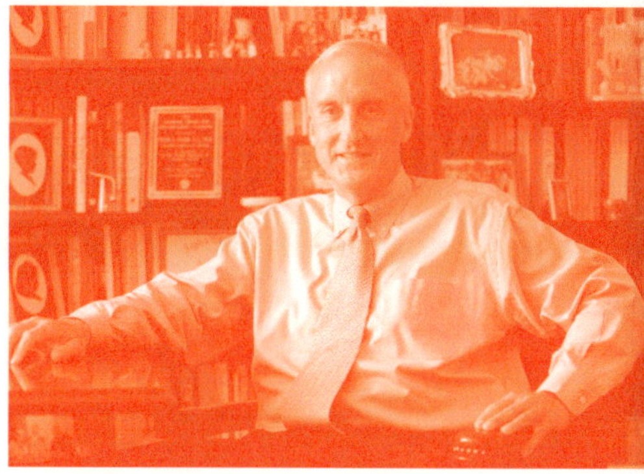
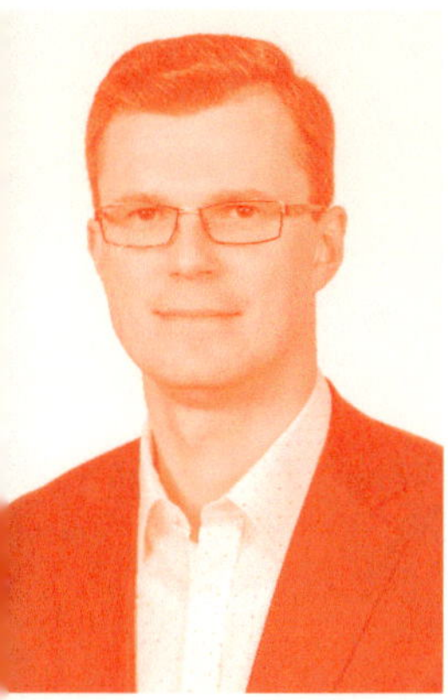
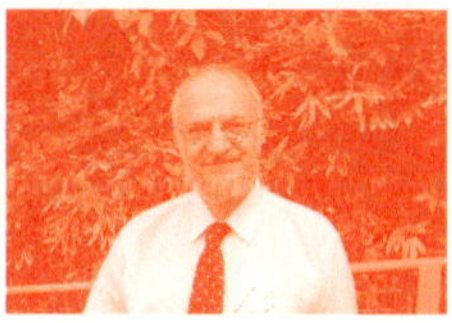
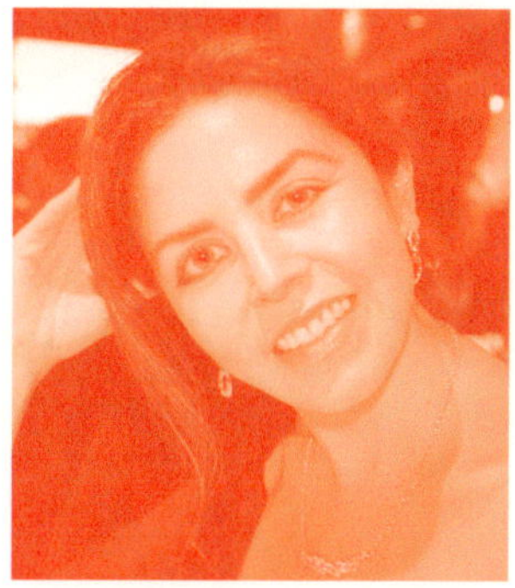

Supporting open minds since 2005

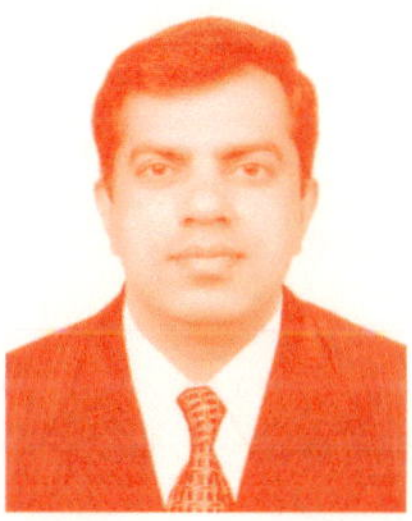
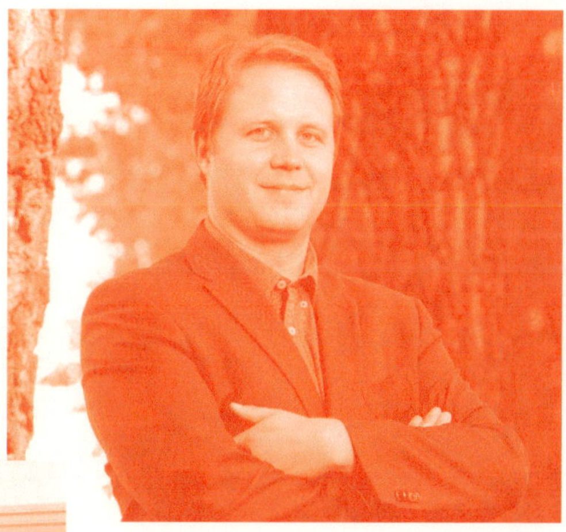
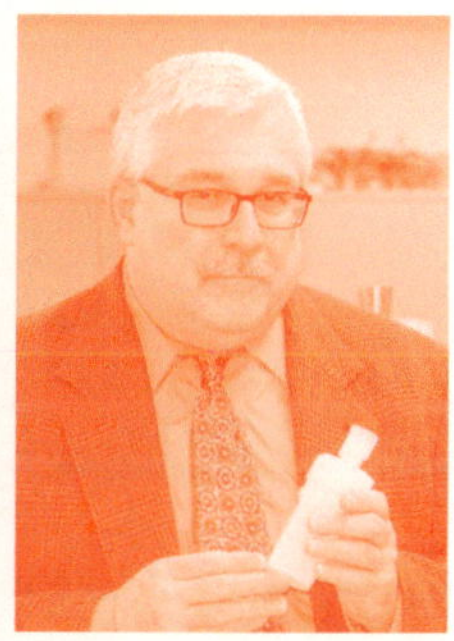
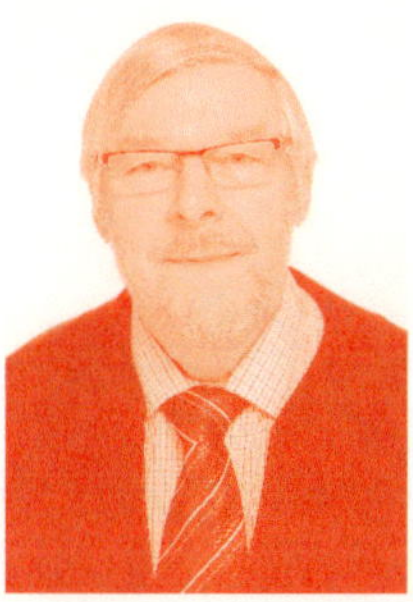
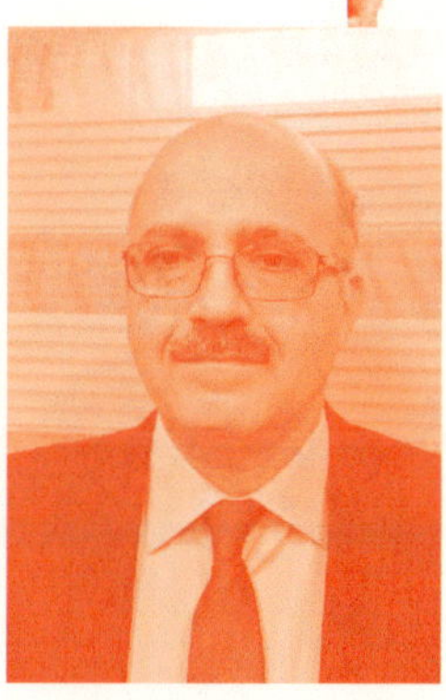
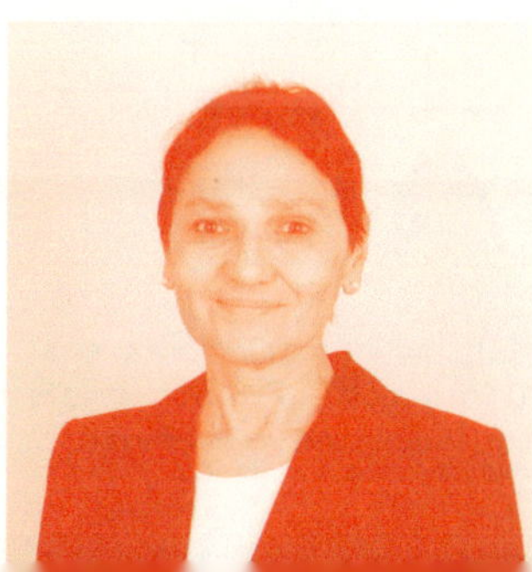
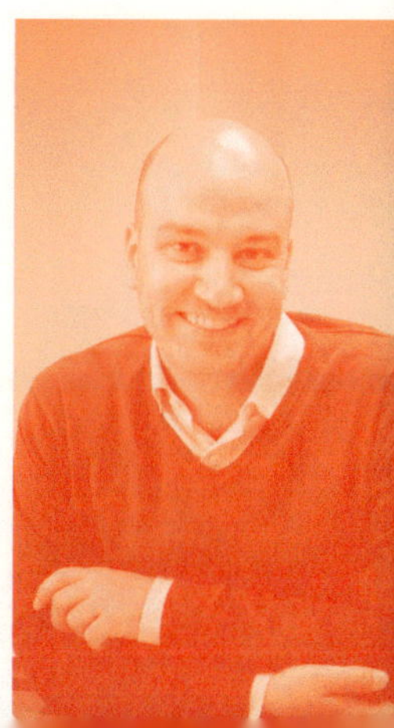

Constipation
http://dx.doi.org/10.5772/intechopen.73896
Edited by Gyula Mózsik

Contributors
Daeyoun Hwang, Charles Lepkowsky, Alexander S. Somwaru, Tika Ram Bhandari, Sudha Shahi, Kenya Kamimura, Masaki Maruyama, Raashid Hamid, Shahid Banday

First published in London, United Kingdom, 2019 by IntechOpen
IntechOpen is the global imprint of INTECHOPEN LIMITED, registered in England and Wales, registration number: 11086078, The Shard, 25th floor, 32 London Bridge Street
London, SE19SG – United Kingdom
Printed in Croatia

British Library Cataloguing-in-Publication Data
A catalogue record for this book is available from the British Library

Additional hard and PDF copies can be obtained from orders@intechopen.com

Constipation
Edited by Gyula Mózsik
p. cm.
Print ISBN 978-1-83881-872-2
Online ISBN 978-1-83881-873-9
eBook (PDF) ISBN 978-1-83881-874-6

For EU product safety concerns:
IN TECH d.o.o., Prolaz Marije Krucifikse Kozulić 3, 51000 Rijeka, Croatia, info@intechopen.com or visit our website at intechopen.com.

Meet the editor

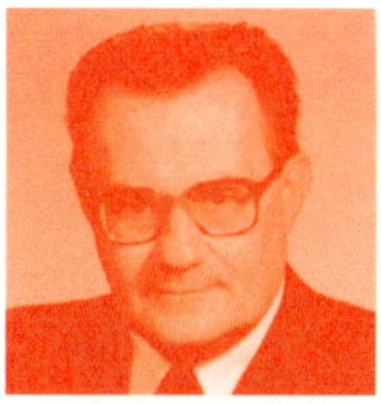

Gyula Mózsik, MD, PhD, ScD, is an emeritus professor of Medicine at the First Department of Medicine, University of Pécs, Hungary. He previously served as head of the department from 1993 to 2003. Dr. Mózsik specializes in medicine, gastroenterology, clinical pharmacology, and clinical nutrition. His research focuses on clinical, pharmacological, biochemical, and molecular studies of the gastrointestinal tract, and innovative studies in new drug production and different foods. He has published 360 peer-reviewed papers, 196 book chapters, 700 abstracts, 19 monographs, and has edited 39 books. He organized 38 national and international congresses/symposiums in Croatia, France, Romania, Italy, the United States, and Japan. He received the Andre Robert award in 2014 from the International Union of Pharmacology, Gastrointestinal Section. Fourteen of Dr. Mózsik's students have been appointed as full professors in Cuba, Egypt, and Hungary.

Contents

Preface

Constipation is not a uniform condition. Although it is a common disorder, there are many different causes. For example, one study found a reverse correlation between the development of constipation and the intake of dietary fibers. It is this multifactorial origin of the problem that makes it difficult to treat. Constipation can result from a number of diseases and disorders, and therefore physicians in different specialties, including gastroenterology, endocrinology, neurology, psychiatry, and so on, may participate in the screening of an individual patient.

This book presents a comprehensive overview of constipation. Chapters cover topics such as prevalence, pathology, diagnosis, imaging, nutrition, and management, among other topics. Future trends and prospects for treatment are also discussed.

During the examinations of patients also a very significant problem is that the possible is that the detailed diseases cover the whole medicine (from the pediatry, to medicine, surgery, traumatology, neurology, psychiratry, nutrition gastroenterology, endocrinology et al. Conseqently many physician partitcipate the screening of one patient.I would like to thank the contributors for their excellent chapters and their help in developing this volume. I am especially thankful for the support I've received from IntechOpen and Ms. Kristina Kardum, Author Service Manager.

Gyula Mózsik, MD,Ph, ScD (med)
First Department of Medicine,
University of Pécs,
Hungary

Chapter 1

Constipation

Tika Ram Bhandari and Sudha Shahi

Abstract

Constipation is a common gastrointestinal (GI) disorder among all age groups. Constipation can be functional or pathological comprising of many etiologies. It can also be classified as acute or chronic; mild to severe. Although in most of the cases it is benign, symptoms can significantly affect the quality of life and cost-related burden for the patient. However, chances of late diagnosis of constipation are high due to a variety of etiologies and variable presentation. Most of the times, it is a great challenge for the clinician to find out the cause of constipation. Healthy lifestyle, especially keeping regular bowel habit, drinking adequate fluid, and the use of high-fiber diet that reduces the viscosity of stool, minimizes intestinal transit time and decreases the chance of constipation. Early diagnosis and management of other underlying factors are important to give relief to the patient from the undue physical and psychological stress.

Keywords: constipation, gastrointestinal disorder, clinical approach, diagnosis, management

1. Introduction

Constipation is a vague term. There is no single definition of it. Constipation is mostly defined by one or more of following symptoms: passage of hard-formed stools or less and dry bowel movements (typically less than three per week), excessive straining, a sense of incomplete bowel evacuation, and excessive time spent on the toilet or in unsuccessful defecation. Nevertheless, even those with regular bowel habits might experience constipation [1, 2]. Similarly, definition of constipation has also been devised according to Rome Criteria (**Table 1**).

Many factors seem to play roles in the causation which when taken care of timely and wisely can create a huge difference. Besides the medical and surgical causes which are mostly unavoidable, food habits and other personal habits are within everyone's control. Healthy lifestyle, consumption of high fiber diet, maintaining adequate hydration and regular bowel habits, careful use of laxatives, and control of medications minimize the problems of constipation.

2. Epidemiology

Constipation is a common condition all around the globe. Worldwide prevalence rates range from 0.7 to 79% with an overall median of 16% and a median of 33.5% among older population [5]. Different surveys have reported the prevalence between 1% and more than 20% in Western populations which can be attributed to different factors [6]. Constipation has been found more prevalent in women than in

Rome II criteria	Rome III for pediatric age group
Adults Two or more of the following for at least 12 weeks (not necessarily consecutive) in the preceding 12 months: • Lumpy or hard stools for >25% of bowel movements • Sensation of anorectal blockage for >25% of bowel movements • Straining during >25% of bowel movements • Sensation of incomplete evacuation for >25% of bowel movements • Manual maneuvers to facilitate >25% of bowel movements (e.g., digital evacuation or support of the pelvic floor) • Loose stools not present and insufficient criteria for irritable bowel syndrome • Less than three bowel movements per week **Infants and children** • Pebble-like, hard stools for a majority of bowel movements for at least 2 weeks • Firm stools $\leq$ 2 times per week for at least 2 weeks • No evidence of structural, endocrine, or metabolic disease	**Child with developmental age < 4 years:** • Less or equal to two defecations per week • At least one incontinence per week after the acquisition of toileting skills • History of painful or hard bowel movements • History of excessive stool retention • History of large-diameter stools that may obstruct the toilet • Presence of a large fecal mass in the rectum • Additional symptoms may include irritability, decreased appetite, and/or early satiety, which may resolve immediately after defecation of a large stool **Child with developmental age $\geq$ 4 years:** • $\leq$ 2 defecations in the toilet per week • At least one episode of fecal incontinence per week • History of retentive posturing or excessive volitional stool retention • History of painful or hard bowel movements • Presence of a large fecal mass in the rectum • History of large-diameter stools that may obstruct the toilet

Table 1.
Rome II criteria [3] and Rome III for pediatric age group [4].

men, in nonwhites than in white persons, in children than in adults, and in elderly than in younger adults. According to the 1996 National Health Interview Survey, about 3 million people in the United States are found to have frequent constipation. Likewise more than 2.5 million visit to physicians, 92,000 hospitalizations, and laxative sales of several hundred million dollars a year in US [7–9]. It has also been stated as a common problem during pregnancy and childbirth [1] According to a study by Jewell DJ and Young G, the prevalence of constipation was estimated to affect 11–38% of pregnancies [10]. To be more specific, constipation is an extremely common disorder in childhood. Up to 25% of all pediatric gastroenterological consultations and 3% of all pediatric outpatient visits are due to constipation. The prevalence of functional constipation at pediatric gastroenterology clinics in secondary or tertiary care hospitals ranged from 1.8 to 13.9% [11]. Studies have shown that 0.7 to 29.6% of children are constipated worldwide. Similarly, 3–5% of pediatric primary care visits and up to 25% of gastroenterology consultations are accounted to constipation. Nearly all childhood constipation is functional, but 5–10% is due to an organic cause [12–16].

Sixty percent of women were found to have constipation at least weekly and more than 90% monthly in a study from Canada. Men had less frequency of constipation and GI symptoms than women. These symptoms were present for more than 10 years in around 60% of women [17]. In the same manner, the prevalence of self-reported constipation was 21% in community-dwelling adults in Australia. The prevalence in Norwegian nursing homes was 23.4%, and 67% while it was found in 50% of institutionalized elderly in a Swedish study. Prevalence in nursing homes in Ireland was 38% [18]. In a study in US elderly above 65 years that reported being constipated, persistent straining was reported by 65%. A study from Finland revealed that 57% of women and 64% of men reported chronic constipation prevalence increased to 79 and 81%, respectively, in a nursing home setting [19–23]. The burden of constipation reflects on work productivity. According to a study by Hunt et al., almost 30% believe that they were less productive at work or at school, 13% missed work or school days, and nearly 10% were late or had to leave work or school because of their symptoms [19].

3. Etiopathogenesis

Constipation is multifactorial most of the times. It can be classified into three broad categories: Normal-transit constipation, slow-transit constipation, and defecatory disorders. In a study of more than 1000 patients with chronic constipation by Mugie Benninga and Di Lorenzo in 2011, normal transit was the most prevalent form (59%) followed by defecatory disorders (25%) and slow transit (13%) and a combination of defecatory disorders and slow transit (3%).

More than one mechanism may contribute to constipation in a patient [5, 24]. Normal-transit constipation is likely due to a perceived difficulty with evacuation or presence of hard stools. Stool traverses at a normal rate in the colon and is responsive to dietary modification alone medications [25]. Dysfunction of the pelvic floor or anal sphincter commonly leads to defecatory disorders. Failure of the rectum to empty effectively may be due to an inability to coordinate the abdominal, rectoanal, and pelvic floor muscles during defecation [26, 27].

Slow-transit constipation occurs most commonly in young women with infrequent bowel movement which occurs by colonic inertia and colonic overactivity mainly due to decreased colonic activity and increased, uncoordinated colon activity. Evacuation disorder is another subtype that occurs due to normal or prolonged colonic transit, but evacuating stools from the rectum are inadequate/difficult [6]. Associated symptoms are an infrequent urge to defecate, bloating, and abdominal pain or discomfort. Symptoms of constipation typically respond to therapy with dietary fiber alone or with the addition of an osmotic laxative [28]. There are a number of factors leading to the above condition that have been listed below [20, 29].

3.1 Causal factors

- Surgical conditions: colorectal tumor and compression form external tumor, diverticulosis, anal fissure, strictures, megacolon, and postsurgical abnormalities
- Metabolic diseases: diabetes mellitus, hypercalcemia, hypokalemia, hypomagnesemia, hypermagnesemia, hyperparathyroidism, hypothyroidism, chronic kidney disease, dehydration, heavy metal poisoning, multiple endocrine neoplasias II, and porphyria
- Gastrointestinal conditions: abscess, anal fissure, fistula irritable bowel syndrome, hemorrhoid, levator ani syndrome, megacolon, proctalgia fugax, rectal prolapse, rectocele, and volvulus
- Musculoskeletal disorder: scleroderma, systemic sclerosis, amyloidosis, and dermatomyositis
- Dietary: eating disorders, dehydration, and low fiber
- Depression and dementia

- Medications
- Others: degenerative joint disease, immobility, cardiac disease, pregnancy, and urinary incontinence

4. Specific associations

4.1 Constipation in children

Children presenting to the emergency department with abdominal pain are most often diagnosed with constipation. Different studies have reported behavior problems higher among children with constipation. Fecal incontinence is a mental disorder that requires psychiatric treatment [30–33]. Other studies, however, have shown that there is a strong association between successful treatment and the reduction of behavior problems suggesting that behavior problems are secondary to the clinical symptoms of constipation [34–36].

4.2 Constipation and morphine

In a study by Joanne Droney et al. in 2007 in cancer patients in morphine, 72% of the patients were found to have mild to severe constipation. Among 53% out of those who were not constipated, 47% were taking laxatives on and off. Of those who said that they were constipated, 73% were already on laxatives, but 27% were not taking any laxatives [37]. Constipation in hospice patients occurs in the majority. About 70–87% opioids account for only 25% of constipation in hospice patients. Persistent constipation correlates with a reduced performance status and not morphine dose. A subgroup of individuals did not require laxatives despite being on higher doses of morphine [38, 39].

4.3 Enuresis association

Yanli Ma et al. in a study from 2016 to 2017 found a positive correlation between constipation (Rome III scores) and frequency of micturition. They also found that constipated children had a higher incidence of severe enuresis and lower incidence of mild-moderate enuresis (68.7 versus 44.6% and 31.3 versus 55.4%) [40].

4.4 Pregnancy and constipation

Hormonal changes during pregnancy, more specifically progesterone rise and serotonin, are responsible for reduced intestinal smooth muscle motility via inhibition of motilin, a smooth muscle stimulant. Similarly relaxin acts on the myometrium and contributes to intestinal gut hypomotility. Another important factor is increased sodium and water reabsorption due to increased aldosterone as a result of increased estrogen and progesterone. This results in hardening of stools [41]. Pregnant women were found to be most prone to developing constipation in the first two trimesters according to a study. In the first and second trimesters, the prevalence of functional constipation ranges between 35 and 39%. Similarly, it is 21 and 17% in the third trimester and puerperium, respectively. Adequate hydration and dietary fiber with or without laxatives are the first line of management. In case of severe or refractory cases, referral is mandatory for further management [42].

Class examples	Examples
5-HT3 receptor antagonists	**Ondansetron**
Analgesics	
Opiates	Morphine
Nonsteroidal anti-inflammatory agents	Ibuprofen
Anticholinergic agents	Belladonna
Tricyclic antidepressants	Amitriptyline, nortriptyline
Antiparkinsonian drugs	Benztropine
Antipsychotics	Chlorpromazine
Antispasmodics	Dicyclomine
Antihistamine	Diphenhydramine
Anticonvulsants	**Carbamazepine**
Antihypertensives	
Calcium channel blockers	Verapamil, nifedipine
Diuretics	Furosemide
Centrally acting	Clonidine
Antiarrhythmics	Amiodarone
Beta-adrenoceptor antagonist	Atenolol
Bile acid sequestrants	**Cholestyramine, Colestipol**
Cation-containing agents	**Aluminum Antacids, Sucralfate**
Iron supplements	**Ferrous sulfate**
Lithium	
Chemotherapy agents	
Vinca alkaloids	Vincristine
Alkylating agents	Cyclophosphamide
Miscellaneous compounds	**Barium sulfate, Oral contraceptives, Polystyrene resins**
Endocrine Medications	**Pamidronateand alendronic acid**
Other antidepressants	**Monoamine oxidase inhibitors**
Other antipsychotics	**Clozapine,haloperidol, risperidone**
Other antiparkinsonian drugs	**Dopamine agonists**
Other antispasmodics	**Mebeverine, peppermint oil**
Sympathomimetics	**Ephedrine, terbutaline**

Table 2.
List of drugs associated with constipation [45].

4.5 Constipation in elderly

Constipation is more frequent among elderly residents of long-term care facilities revealed by a study from the United States in persons older than 65 years. There are intrinsic changes, reduced number of neurons in myenteric plexus, and reduction in the amplitude of inhibitory nerve input to circular muscle layer of colon causing constipation in the elderly that has been found in the study of colonic physiology [43, 44].

4.6 Medications associated with constipation

Many groups of drugs have been found to be strong correlated with constipation, highest for calcium channel blockers, and least for antiarrhythmics (**Table 2**).

5. Symptoms and signs of constipation

Constipation basically is a subjective condition. This is why the most important tool for diagnosis of constipation mostly depends upon the clinical history. The signs and symptoms common for both childhood and adult constipation are Irregular bowel activity with excessive foul-smelling flatulence and stools with irregular texture. Sometimes patients may present with history of passage of small pellets or less frequent large amount of stools and painful defecation. Withholding or straining at stools, soiling or overflow. Abdominal distension or discomfort, decreased appetite, easy fatigability, and irritable mood are few other symptoms.

6. Diagnosis and diagnostic approaches

Diagnosis mostly depends upon clinical history aided by radiological examination and blood examination to rule out underlying conditions: a thorough history taking and physical examination can rule out most secondary causes of constipation.

6.1 Steps of evaluation

6.1.1 The clinical history and physical examination

Assessment of clinical criteria, presence of risk factors, and identification of alarming features indicate the need for colonoscopy and/or radiological examination to rule out secondary causes [46, 47]. Digital rectal examination and proctological examination may help to identify surgical causes of constipation. A careful rectal examination should be performed in every patient with constipation and is often the most revealing part of the clinical evaluation. A number of criteria have been devised by different studies for the evaluation of constipation that have been approved in the clinical practice which are as shown below.

6.1.1.1 Classic Lowa criteria

Pediatric constipation is defined whenever presence of at least two of the following criteria [48]:

- Two or more encopresis episodes per week
- Defecation frequency less than 3 times per week
- Periodic passage of very large amounts of stool once every 7–30 days (the criterion of a large amount of stool is satisfied if it is estimated to be twice the standard amount of stool, shown in a clay model, or if stools are so large that they clog the toilet).

Solitary encopresis is defined in a child older than 4 years of age:

- Two or more encopresis episodes per week
- Defecation frequency equal or more than 3 times per week

No passage of very large amounts of stool.

6.1.1.2 Paris consensus on childhood constipation terminology (PACCT criteria)

Chronic constipation is caused by the occurrence of two or more of the following characteristics during the preceding 8 weeks [49]:

- Fewer than three bowel movements per week
- More than one episode of fecal incontinence per week
- Large stools in the rectum or palpable on abdominal examination
- Passage of large-diameter stools that may obstruct the toilet
- Display of retentive posturing and withholding behaviors
- Painful defecation

6.1.2 Investigations

Fecal, radiological, or endoscopic examinations are not routinely indicated in case where severe symptoms are absent. Sigmoidoscopy is usually sufficient in patients without severe symptoms and those under 50 years of age. Adults more than 50 years of age are entitled to colonoscopy or both sigmoidoscopy and barium-enema examination to rule out colorectal carcinoma.

6.1.3 Blood tests

Electrolyte imbalances, metabolic disorders, endocrine disorders, and parasitological infestation can be can be ruled out by blood test. These examinations should be ordered mainly in clinically suspicious cases.

6.1.4 Barium defecography

Barium defecography is an X-ray test where a thick paste containing barium is placed into the rectum. It determines whether there are any abnormalities in the pelvic floor. It is recommended to identify colorectal diseases (diverticular disease, neoplasia, and megacolon).

6.1.5 Anorectal manometry

This test measures the pressure in anal canal when patient pushes during a bowel movement. This test is recommended in cases refractory to medical treatment. The main aim is to rule out diseases like aganglionosis and psychogenic megacolon. It provides information about the rectoanal inhibitory reflex, the musculature tone of the internal and external sphincters, and the rectal sensitivity, capacity, and complacency.

6.1.6 Videodefecography, magnetic resonance defecography, or echodefecography

Videodefecography is the radiological study of evacuatory dynamics. It is useful in the study of abnormalities such as rectocele, intussusception, enterocele, sigmoidocele, anismus, and paradoxical contraction of the puborectalis muscle. Recent literature suggest video defecography using only video recording without radiography because of its high radiation exposure, whereas others have chosen magnetic resonance defecography or echodefecography, without the use of ionizing radiation.

6.1.7 The colonic transit time (CTT) examination

A capsule containing radiopaque markers is swallowed and an abdominal radiography is taken 5 days later. With this, the identification of three types of patterns in patients can be done; in normal transit time, patients eliminate 80% of the markers by the fifth day. In slow transit, more than 20% of the marker is retained by the fifth day, distributed throughout the colon, and in those with bowel obstruction, they retain more than 20% of the markers on the fifth day which remains accumulated in the rectosigmoid region. Though it is a noninvasive test, there is exposure to radiation even in low doses. CTT may be recommended to assess the success of clinical or surgical treatment of chronic constipation.

6.1.8 Balloon expulsion test

A balloon filled with water (50–60 mL) is positioned in the rectal ampulla. If expulsion is achieved by patient, pelvic floor dysfunction may be excluded. It has been recommended by many constipation evaluation guidelines.

6.1.9 Electromyography of the anal sphincter (EMG)

Small electrical sensors are placed in the anal canal to record the electrical activity of sphincter muscles during voluntary contraction, at rest, and with coughing and evacuatory effort.

6.1.10 Hydrogen breath test

It is recommended for assessing the orocecal transit time. It aids to differentiate dysmotility of the gastrointestinal tract (superior and inferior) from isolated colonic inertia. It is recommended for serious and refractory cases of colonic inertia, prior to the indication of a colectomy. Similarly a number of criteria have been devised by different studies for the evaluation of constipation.

7. Management of constipation

7.1 Lifestyle modifications

Dehydration and decrease in physical activity are found to worsen so different studies recommend adequate hydration and increase in physical activity [50].

High fiber diet is found to be beneficial for constipation. The ideal amount is 25–35 g per day. Fiber adds bulk to stools and makes bowel movements soft or firm. To improve compliance with treatment, patients should be instructed to increase their dietary fiber intake gradually to 20–25 g per day over a period of 1–2 weeks. If this approach is not effective, commercially packaged fiber supplements should be tried. Regular bowel habits, careful use of laxatives, and control of medications including dosage and timing are also effective for constipation.

7.2 Medications commonly used for constipation

7.2.1 Laxatives

7.2.1.1 Bulk laxative

The medications used for constipation are stated below in order [1].
Psyllium (Metamucil, Perdiem, and Fiberall)

- Natural fiber should be taken with plenty of water to avoid intestinal obstruction; allergic reactions such as anaphylaxis and asthma are rare; titrate up to 20 g.

Methylcellulose (Citrucel)

- Semisynthetic cellulose fiber that is relatively resistant to colonic bacterial degradation; titrate up to 20 g

Polycarbophil (FiberCon, Equalactin, and Konsyl)

- Synthetic fiber of polymer of acrylic acid, resistant to bacterial degradation; titrate up to 20 g

7.2.1.2 Osmotic laxative

This draws water into the intestines along osmotic gradient.
Magnesium hydroxide (Phillips' Milk of Magnesia); 15–30 ml once or twice.
Magnesium citrate (Evac-Q-Mag); 150–300 ml as needed.
Sodium phosphate (Fleet Enema, Fleet Phospho-Soda, Visicol); 10–25 ml with 12 oz. (360 ml) of water as needed.

7.2.1.3 Poorly absorbed sugar

Lactulose (Cephulac, Chronulac, and Duphalac);
Synthetic disaccharide; 15–30 ml once or twice a day.

7.2.1.4 Stimulant laxative

Stimulates intestinal motility or secretion.
Anthraquinones.
Cascara sagrada (Coleman, Sagrada-lax): 325 mg (or 5 ml) daily.
Senna (Senokot, Ex-Lax): 187 mg daily.
Castor oil (Purge, Neoloid, Emulsoil): 15–30 ml daily.
Bisacodyl (Dulcolax, Correctol): 5–10 mg every night.
Sodium picosulfate (Lubrilax, Sur-Lax): 5–15 mg every night.

7.2.1.5 Stool softener

Docusate sodium (Colace, Regulax SS, Surfak): 100 mg twice a day.
Mineral oil (Fleet Mineral Oil): 5–15 ml orally every night.

Phosphate enema (Fleet Enema): 120 ml daily.
Mineral oil retention enema (Fleet Mineral Oil Enema): 100 ml daily.
Tap-water enema: 500 ml daily.
Soapsuds enema: 1500 ml daily.
Glycerin bisacodyl suppository: 10 mg daily.

7.2.2 Cholinergic agent

Bethanechol (Urecholine): 10 mg daily.

7.2.3 Miscellaneous

Colchicine (Colsalide): 0.6 mg three times a day.
Misoprostol (Cytotec): 600–2400 μg daily.

7.2.4 Prokinetic agent

Tegaserod is a colonic prokinetic agent that improves stool consistency and frequency in women with irritable bowel syndrome characterized by constipation.
5-HT4 receptor agonists* Cisapride (Propulsid): 10–20 mg four times a day.
Tegaserod (Zelnorm): 6 mg, twice a day.

7.2.5 Emerging drugs

Velusetrag and Naronapride (5-HT4 receptor agonists), Pumosetrag (5-HT3 receptor agonist) and few other drugs like plecanatide (colonic secretagogue), methylnaltrexone (opioid receptor antagonist), elobixibat (prokinetic secretagogue), and alvimopan (opioid receptor antagonist) are the few emerging drugs for management of constipation [51].

7.3 Surgical management

Those patients who do not benefit from conservative treatment and without intestinal obstruction may profit from subtotal colectomy with ileorectal anastomosis. Refractory constipation may have good results from total colonic resection and ileorectostomy in a patient without defecatory disorder. A systematic review of 32 studies reported satisfactory results post colectomy ranging between 39 and 100% of patients. Few complications like diarrhea, incontinence, and intestinal obstructions were reported. Similarly, in some studies, it was revealed that laparoscopic subtotal colectomy was equally effective in those who were suitable for colonic resection [52–54].

7.4 Miscellaneous

7.4.1 Biofeedback

This represents a behavioral treatment. Patients are trained regarding physiological mechanisms of defecation. The use of their diaphragms and abdominal and pelvic floor muscles for evacuation is emphasized. Sensory retraining is also given [30]. Auditory or visual response, or both, on the functioning and coordination of their anal sphincter and pelvic floor muscles is provided to patients. Balloon or silicon-filled artificial stool, which is also termed as "freedom," can be used as biofeedback with more focus to normal coordination for successful defecation [1]. Educating the patients and a good rapport between the physician and the patients are keys to successful biofeedback. Different studies on biofeedback treatment have reported an overall success rate of 67%. Nevertheless, adequate data regarding the successful practice of biofeedback are still missing [55–57].

7.4.2 Abdominal massage

According to different studies, there is a positive influence of abdominal massage in constipation [58–60].

7.4.3 Botulinum type A toxin

Injection of botulinum type A toxin into the puborectalis muscle may be beneficial in the treatment of defecatory disorders revealed by some studies. However, no controlled trials have been done till date, so this method is not suggested [61].

8. Conclusions

Constipation is a very common problem worldwide that presents as a subtle disease yet can have relenting effects in a patient's life. There are a number of preventable risk factors, like food habit and personal habits, causing constipation; taking care of them on time can play an important role in minimizing their effects which in turn minimizes the socioeconomic burden of constipation significantly. Apart from that, the early diagnosis and management of other underlying factors are important to give relief to the patient from the undue physical and psychological stress.

Conflict of interest

All authors declare that there is no conflict of interest.

Author details

Tika Ram Bhandari[1,2,3]* and Sudha Shahi[4]

1 Department of General Surgery, People's Dental College and Hospital, Kathmandu, Nepal

2 Formerly Department of Surgery, Institute of Medicine, Tribhuvan University Teaching Hospital, Kathmandu, Nepal

3 Formerly Department of Surgery, Universal College of Medical Sciences, Bhairahawa, Nepal

4 Department of Otorhinolaryngology Head and Neck Surgery, National Academy of Medical Sciences, Bir Hospital, Kathmandu, Nepal

*Address all correspondence to: tikanmc@gmail.com

References

[1] Lembo A, Camilleri M. Current concepts chronic constipation. The New England Journal of Medicine. 2003; **349**(14):1360-1368

[2] NICE Guidelines: Constipation in children. Internet communication. 2010. http://www.nice.org.uk/guidance/CG99

[3] Thompson WG, Longstreth GF, Drossman DA, Heaton KW, Irvine EJ, Muller-Lissner SA. Functional bowel disorders and functional abdominal pain. Gut. 1999;**45**(2):II-43-II-47

[4] Longstreth GF et al. Functional Bowel Disorders - Gastroenterology;**130** (5):1480-1491

[5] Mugie SM, Bennings MA, Di Lorenzo C. Epidemiology of constipation in children and adults: A systematic review. Best Practice & Research: Clinical Obstetrics & Gynaecology. 2011;**25**(1):3

[6] Lindberg G, Hamid SS, Malfertheiner P, Thomsen OO, Fernandez LB, Garisch J, et al. World gastroenterology organisation global guideline: Constipation—A global perspective. Journal of Gastroenterology. 2011;**45**(6):483

[7] Sonnenberg A, Koch TR. Physician visits in the United States for constipation: 1958 to 1986. Digestive Diseases and Sciences. 1989;**34**:606-611

[8] Heaton KW, Radvan J, Cripps H, Mountford(women) 5RA, Braddon FE, Hughes AO. Defecation frequency and timing, and stool form in the general population: A prospective study. Gut. 1992;**33**:818-824

[9] Johanson JF, Sonnenberg A, Koch TR. (whites) clinical epidemiology of chronic constipation. Journal of Clinical Gastroenterology. 1989;**11**:525-536

[10] Jewell DJ, Young G. Interventions for treating constipation in pregnancy. Cochrane Database of Systematic Reviews. 2001;(2):CD001142

[11] Tabbers MM, Dilorenzo C, Berger MY, et al. Evaluation and treatment of functional constipation in infants and children: Evidence-based recommendations from ESPGHAN and NASPGHAN. Journal of Pediatric Gastroenterology and Nutrition. 2014; **58**(2):265-281

[12] Milla PJ. Endothelins, pseudo-obstruction and Hirschsprung's disease. Gut. 1999;**44**:148-149

[13] Chang SH, Park KY, Kang SK, Kang KS, Na SY, Yang HR, et al. Prevalence, clinical characteristics, and management of functional constipation at pediatric gastroenterology clinics. Journal of Korean Medical Science. 2013;**28**(9): 1356-1361

[14] Higgins PD, Johanson JF. Epidemiology of constipation in North America: A systematic review. The American Journal of Gastroenterology. 2004;**99**:750-759

[15] Johanson JF, Kralstein J. Chronic constipation: A survey of the patient perspective. Alimentary Pharmacology & Therapeutics. 2007;**25**:599-608

[16] Caperell K, Pitetti R, Cross KP. Race and acute abdominal pain in the pediatric emergency department. Pediatrics. 2013;**131**(6):1098-10106

[17] Di Lorenzo C. Childhood constipation: Finally some hard data about hard stools! The Journal of Pediatrics. 2000;**136**(1):4

[18] Youssef NN, Di Lorenzo C. Childhood constipation: Evaluation and

treatment. Journal of Clinical Gastroenterology. 2001;**33**(3):199-205

[19] Hunt RH, Dhaliwal S, Tougas G, Pedro C, Labbé J-F, Paul H, et al. Prevalence, impact, and attitudes toward lower gastrointestinal dysmotility and sensory symptoms, and their treatment in Canada: A descriptive study. Canadian Journal of Gastroenterology. 2007;**21**(1):31-37

[20] Russell B, Buswell M, Norton C, Malone JR, Harari D, Harwood R, et al. Supporting people living with dementia and fecal incontinence. British Journal of Community Nursing. 2017;**22**(3): 110-114

[21] Klaus JH, Nardin VD, Paludo J, Scherer F, Bosco SM. The prevalence and factors associated with constipation in elderly residents of long-stay institutions. Revista Brasileira de Geriatria e Gerontologia. 2015;**18**(4): 835-843

[22] Coyne KS, Cash B, Kopp Z, et al. The prevalence of chronic constipation and fecal incontinence among men and women with symptoms of overactive bladder. BJU International. 2011;**107**: 254-261

[23] Kinnunen A. Study of constipation in a geriatric hospital, day hospital, old people's home and at home. Aging (Milano). 1991;**3**:161-170

[24] Nyam DC, Pemberton JH, Ilstrup DM, Rath DM. Long-term results of surgery for chronic constipation. Diseases of the Colon and Rectum. 1997; **40**:273-279. [Erratum, Dis Colon Rectum 1997;**40**:529]

[25] Ashraf W, Park F, Lof J, Quigley EM. An examination of the reliability of reported stool frequency in the diagnosis of idiopathic constipation. The American Journal of Gastroenterology. 1996;**91**:26-32

[26] Camilleri M, Thompson WG, Fleshman JW, Pemberton JH. Clinical management of intractable constipation. Annals of Internal Medicine. 1994;**121**: 520-528

[27] Rao SS, Welcher KD, Leistikow JS. Obstructive defecation: A failure of rectoanal coordination. The American Journal of Gastroenterology. 1998;**93**: 1042-1050

[28] Preston DM, Lennard-Jones JE. Severe chronic constipation of young women: 'Idiopathic slow transit constipation'. Gut. 1986;**27**:41-48

[29] Bouras EP, Tangalos EG. Chronic constipation in the elderly. Gastroenterology Clinics of North America. 2009;**38**:463-480

[30] Elkhayat HA, Shehata MH, Nada A, Deifalla SM, Ammar MS. Impact of constipation on psychosocial functioning and quality of life of children: A cross-sectional study. Egyptian Pediatric Association Gazette. 2016;**64**(3):136-141

[31] van Dijk M, Benninga MA, Grootenhuis MA, Onland-van Nieuwenhuizen AM, Last BF. Chronic childhood constipation: A review of the literature and the introduction of a protocolized behavioral intervention program. Patient Education and Counseling. 2007;**67**(1–2):63-77

[32] Kianifar H, Hebrani P, Behdani F, Dadpour MN, Karami H, Mehdizadeh A. Quality of life and psychiatric comorbidity in children and adolescents with functional constipation: A case-control study. Govaresh. 2016;**21**(3):193-198

[33] Bemporad JR, Kresch RA, Asnes R, Wilson A. Chronic neurotic encopresis as a paradigm of a multifactorial psychiatric disorder. The Journal of Nervous and Mental Disease. 1978; **166**(7):472-479

[34] Nolan T, Debelle G, Oberklaid F, Coffey C. Randomised trial of laxatives in treatment of childhood encopresis. Lancet. 1991;**338**(8766):523-527

[35] Young MH, Brennen LC, Baker RD, Baker SS. Functional encopresis: Symptom reduction and behavioral improvement. Journal of Developmental and Behavioral Pediatrics. 1995;**16**(4): 226-232

[36] van der Plas RN, Benninga MA, Redekop WK, Taminiau JA, Buller HA. Randomized trial of biofeedback training for encopresis. Archives of Disease in Childhood. 1996;**75**(5): 367-373

[37] Droney J Ross J, Gretton S, Welsh K, Sato H, Riley J. Constipation in cancer patients on morphine. Supportive Care in Cancer. 2008;**16**(5):453-459

[38] Fallon MT, Hanks GW. Morphine, constipation and performance status in advanced cancer patients. Palliative Medicine. 1999;**13**(2):159-160

[39] Sykes NP. The relationship between opioid use and laxative use in terminally ill cancer patients. Palliative Medicine. 1998;**12**(5):375-382

[40] Ma Y, Shen Y, Liu X. Functional constipation and bladder capacity and severity of enuresis in children: A correlation study. International Journal of Clinical and Experimental Medicine. 2018;**11**(2):806-811

[41] Verghese TS, Futaba K, Latthe P. Constipation in pregnancy. The Obstetrician and Gynaecologist. 2015; **17**(20):111-115

[42] Derbyshire E, Davies J, Costarelli V, Dettmar P. Diet, physical inactivity and the prevalence of constipation throughout and after pregnancy. Maternal & Child Nutrition. 2006;**2**: 127-134

[43] Fragakis A, Zhou J, Mannan H, Ho V. Association between drug usage and constipation in the elderly population of greater Western Sydney Australia. International Journal of Environmental Research and Public Health. 2018;**15**(2): 226

[44] Gallegos-Orozco JF, Foxx-Orenstein SSM, Stoa JM. Chronic constipation in the elderly. The American Journal of Gastroenterology. 2012;**107**:18-25

[45] Bharucha AE, Pemberton JH, Locke GR. American gastroenterological association technical review on constipation. Gastroenterology. 2013; **144**(1):218-238

[46] Drossman DA. Functional gastrointestinal disorders: History, pathophysiology, clinical features, and Rome IV. Gastroenterology. 2016;**150**: 1262-1279

[47] Ternent CA, Bastawrous AL, Morin NA, Ellis CN, Hyman NH, Buie WD. Practice parameters for the evaluation and management of constipation. Diseases of the Colon and Rectum. 2007; **50**(12):2013-2022

[48] Loening-Baucke V. Functional faecal retention with encopresis in childhood. Journal of Pediatric Gastroenterology and Nutrition. 2004; **38**:79-84

[49] Benninga M, Candy DC, Catto-Smith AG, Clayden G, Loening-Baucke V, Di Lorenzo C, et al. The Paris consensus on childhood constipation terminology (PACCT) group. Journal of Pediatric Gastroenterology and Nutrition. 2005;**40**:273-275

[50] Chua HC, Nieh CC. The Effect of Lifestyle Modification in Treatment of Constipation in Older Adult. MedCrave Group LLC; 2016

[51] Basilisco G, Coletta M. Chronic constipation: A critical review. Digestive and Liver Disease. 2013;**45**:886-888

[52] Knowles CH, Scott M, Lunniss PJ. Outcome of colectomy for slow transit constipation. Annals of Surgery. 1999; **230**:627-638

[53] Redmond JM, Smith GW, Barofsky I, Ratych RE, Goldsborough DC, Schuster MM. Physiological tests to predict long-term outcome of total abdominal colectomy for intractable constipation. The American Journal of Gastroenterology. 1995;**90**: 748-753

[54] Young-Fadok TM. Raising the bar: Laparoscopic resection of colorectal cancer. Surgical Endoscopy. 2001;**15**: 911-912

[55] Pelsang RE, Rao SS, Welcher K. FECOM: A new artificial stool for evaluating defecation. The American Journal of Gastroenterology. 1999;**94**: 183-186

[56] Koutsomanis D, Lennard-Jones JE, Roy AJ, Kamm MA. Controlled randomised trial of visual biofeedback versus muscle training without a visual display for intractable constipation. Gut. 1995;**37**:95-99

[57] Enck P. Biofeedback training in disordered defecation: A critical review. Digestive Diseases and Sciences. 1993; **38**:1953-60.7:95-9

[58] Ayas S, Leblebici B, Sozay S, Bayramoglu M, Niron EA. The effect of abdominal massage on bowel function in patients with spinal cord injury. American Journal of Physical Medicine & Rehabilitation. 2006;**85**(12):951-955

[59] Harrington KL, Haskvitz EM. Managing a patient's constipation with physical therapy. Physical Therapy. 2006;**86**(11):1511-1519

[60] Holey LA, Lawler H. The effects of classical massage and connective tissue manipulation on bowel function. British Journal of Therapy and Rehabilitation. 1995;**2**(11):627-631

[61] Ron Y, Avni Y, Lukovetski A, et al. Botulinum toxin type-a in the therapy of patients with anismus. Diseases of the Colon and Rectum. 2001;**44**:1821-1826

Chapter 2

Management of Pediatric Constipation

Raashid Hamid and Shazada Shahid Banday

Abstract

Constipation is a common problem in children. It accounts for 20–30% of pediatric outdoor office. It is common in both rich and poor countries despite the belief that developing countries consume food rich in fiber. Normal bowel movement in breastfed babies may range from several times a day to once in every 10 days. Constipation can be both functional and pathological. Functional constipation has no underlying cause and is the most common type of constipation found in children. My main focus will be on this common type of constipation. In functional constipation routine, digital rectal examination is not recommended unless impaction is suspected. Abdominal radiography is recommended only in equivocal clinical examination or if impaction is suspected and examination not conclusive. Dietary and behavior modifications, toilet training, and parent education are important in the management of functional constipation. Initial management of functional constipation includes disimpaction of stools. Lactulose is safe in all age groups. Polyethylene glycol is more effective than lactulose but is costly. Maintenance therapy may take some time till constipation improves. Some rare situations such as refractory and slow transient constipation are also discussed in this chapter.

Keywords: functional constipation, laxatives, children

1. Introduction

Constipation in children is a common problem and accounts for up to 25% of pediatric clinical consultation [1]. The most common cause of constipation is functional (without any organic etiology or anatomical malformation), with an estimated prevalence of 3% worldwide. Infants on an average pass four stools per day in the first day of life, which gradually decreases to an average of 1.7 stools per day at 2 years of age and 1.2 stools per day at 4 years of age [2]. Evidence suggests that dietary, lifestyle, cognitive, emotional/behavioral, and broader psychosocial factors may all play a role in the etiology, maintenance, and clinically effective treatment of functional GI disorders. Constipated children have more outpatient and emergency department visits for abdominal pain, and their overall annual medical cost is approximately twice as much as that of children without constipation. Diagnosis of functional constipation requires a careful history and thorough physical examination. Management includes initial disimpaction followed by maintenance therapy with dietary modification, toilet training, and oral laxative. Laxatives may be needed for several months and sometimes years [3]. Noncompliance to laxative is the commonest cause of recurrence. Refractory constipation is defined as nonresponse to optimal treatment for at least 3 months. This form of constipation may be diagnosed by colon transit time (CTT) study, which can be done by radio-opaque markers and by radionuclide scintigraphy. Antegrade continence enema is an option in patients with optimal CTT. Children with constipation having warning signs need further evaluation in the form of anorectal manometry barium/contrast enema and sometimes rectal biopsy. Absence of ganglion cells on rectal biopsy suggests Hirschsprung's disease requiring surgical treatment [4].

2. Definition of constipation

Functional constipation is defined as presence of two or more of the following ROME III criteria in the absence of any organic etiology, and the duration of constipation should at least be 1 month in children <4 years of age, and at least once per week for at least 2 months in children ≥4 years of age [5] (**Table 1**).

Child with age < 4 years	Child with age ≥ 4 years
• ≤2 defecations/week	• ≤2 defecations in the toilet per week
• One episode of incontinence per week after	• One episode of fecal incontinence per week
• Excessive stool retention	• Retentive posturing or excessive volitional stool retention
• Painful or hard bowel movements	• Painful or hard bowel movements
• Presence of a large fecal mass in the rectum	• Large fecal mass in the rectum
• Large-diameter stools that may obstruct the toilet	• Large-diameter stools that may obstruct the toilet

Table 1.
Diagnostic criteria for functional constipation in children.

3. Etiology and pathogenesis of constipation

Disruption of the normal physiology leads to constipation. Constipation may result from impaired propulsion of stools, sensation of rectum, and rectal outlet obstruction [6]. Disruption of the normal physiology leads to constipation. Constipation may, result from impaired propulsion of stools, sensation of rectum, rectal outlet obstruction. Conditions that lead to impaired propulsion are metabolic abnormalities such as hypo/hypercalcemia, hypothyroidism, cystic fibrosis, celiac disease, and genetic predisposition. Use of narcotics, psychotropics, and anticholinergic defective/impaired sensation may occur in spinal cord abnormalities or secondary sensory impairment due to megarectum from chronic fecal retention. Other anatomical and pathological causes of constipation include Hirschsprung's disease, imperforate anus, pelvic or sacral mass, anal or colonic stricture, anteriorly displaced anus or Functional as in intentional fecal retention, and pelvic floor dyssynergia.

Breastfed infants produce more frequent and larger stools than those fed standard infant formula until food is introduced at 5 months of age. Bowel movement frequency decreases with age. Stool production occurs more often in the first month of life and may be attributed to immaturity of the gastrointestinal tract. The passage of hard stool are perceived as painful leading to stool withholding, as the child becomes afraid to defecate. Furthermore, withholding creates a cycle of more pain on defecating (**Figure 1**). Signs of withholding behavior include arching the back, stiffening the legs, and unusual postures/crossing of legs in older children [7]. Parents may misinterpret withholding as straining or an attempt to defecate.

It can be challenging for some parents to toilet train their children. Research supports that stool toileting refusal occurs in 1 of every 5 children. This leads to stool withholding behavior and incontinence [8]. Functional constipation is at times associated with autism and attention-deficit hyperactivity disorder (ADHD). However, the literature indicates that the rate of constipation does not differ significantly between children with or without ADHD [9]. Other causes diet changes such as the introduction of solids or cow's milk, illness, and change in routine. In some situations, children defer the defecation by playing, operating computers, watching

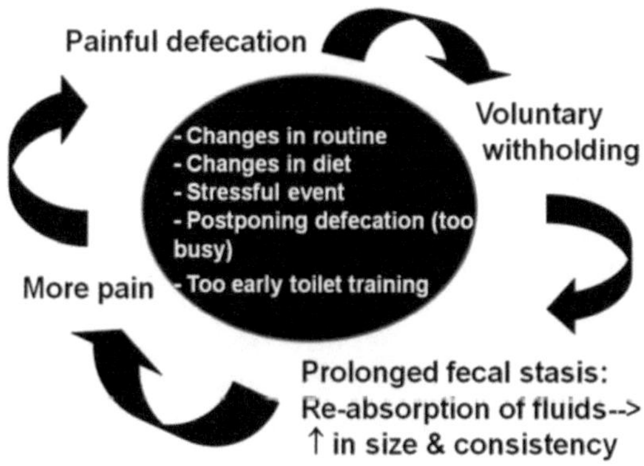

Figure 1.
Viscous circle of constipation and pain. Painful defecation leads to voluntary withholding behavior and prolonged fecal stasis (stools becomes harder and larger). Passage of hard stools leads to more pain due to fissures which further aggravates constipation.

a. Anal achalasia
b. Colonic inertia
c. Anatomic malformations
d. Imperforate anus
e. Anal stenosis
f. Celiac disease
g. HSD
h. Dietary protein allergy
i. Vitamin D intoxication
j. Cystic fibrosis
k. Pelvic mass (sacrococcygeal teratoma)
l. Spinal cord anomalies, trauma, tethered cord
m. Abnormal abdominal musculature (prune belly, gastroschisis, Down syndrome)
n. Hypothyroidism, hypercalcemia, hypokalemia
o. Diabetes mellitus
p. Opiates, anticholinergics
q. Pseudo-obstruction (visceral neuropathies, myopathies, mesenchymopathies)
r. Multiple endocrine neoplasia type 2B

Table 2.
Causes of constipation in infants/toddlers and children/adolescents.

television, and nonavailability/unhygienic conditions of the toilet rooms. Moreover some children remain in hurry and do not spend enough time completely emptying the rectum of stool. Common pathological causes of constipation in childhood include, Hirschsprung's disease, myopathy, congenital anomalies like anal stenosis, anteriorly located anus, spinal cord anomalies (meningomyelocele, myelomalacia, spina bifida), hypothyroidism, hypercalcemia, cerebral palsy, and mental retardation. Some drugs causing constipation include anticonvulsants, antipsychotic, codeine containing antidiarrheal [10] (**Table 2**).

4. Sequelae of constipation

Fecal retention contributes to dysfunctional voiding, vesicoureteral reflux, and urinary tract infections. Increased stool in the rectum can cause abnormal bladder pressure and function. Urinary tract infections and enuresis occur in 30% of constipated children [11]. Some patients with constipation present as abdominal pain, obstruction, loss of apetite, and poor school attendance.

5. Evaluation of constipation

A thorough history and examination is very essential part of complete evaluation of a child with constipation. Important information includes any history of delayed passage of meconium, duration of constipation, the frequency of bowel movements, the consistency and size of the stools, painful defecation, bleeding per rectum (blood present in the stool or the toilet paper), abdominal pain. Identification of alarm signs favors organic diseases, and these signs are given in **Table 3** [13].

The current evidence-based recommendations do not support digital examination of the anorectum, unless the diagnosis of functional constipation is uncertain, alarm signs are present, or there is intractable constipation. Abdominal radiograph is only recommended if fecal impaction is suspected clinically and physical examination is unreliable or not possible. Routine laboratory tests for hypothyroid, celiac disease, or hypercalcemia are not indicated, unless alarm symptoms are present [13] (**Table 4**).

Some children have a history of irregular bowel movements without clear history of constipation, and in these cases, colonic transit time (CTT) with radiopaque markers study can be useful. The history obtained may also be not as clear and in these patients, an evaluation can be helpful [14]. The CTT study provides objective evaluation of bowel movement.

Younger the infant (less than 6 months) more are the chances of an organic etiology for constipation. Hirschsprung's disease (HSD) must be suspected in infants with history delayed passage of meconium (more than 48 h after birth), constipation since birth, recurrent abdominal distention and enterocolitis. In infants, neonated HSD can present as enterocolitis, a potentially fatal complication that presents as fever, abdominal distension, and explosive, bloody diarrhea. Patients with suspected Hirschsprung's disease should be referred to a pediatric surgeon. On examination, the position (anteriorly displaced anus) and patency of the anus should be assessed. Spinal examination should be done for spina bifida and tethered cord [13, 15].

Further evaluation is indicated in older children with red flags or with intractable constipation despite strict adherence to therapy. Laboratory studies should

1. Distented abdomen
2. Absent lumbosacral curve
3. Pilonidal sinus/dimple covered by a tuft of hair
4. Midline pigmentary abnormalities of the lower spine
5. Sacral agenesis
6. Flat buttocks
7. Anteriorly displaced anus
8. Patulous anus
9. Tight, empty rectum in presence of palpable abdominal fecal mass
10. Gush of liquid stool and air from rectum on withdrawal of finger
11. Occult blood in stool
12. Absent anal wink
13. Absent cremasteric reflex
14. Decreased lower limb tone and/or strength
15. Absence or delay in relaxation phase of lower extremity deep tendon reflex
16. Failure to thrive

Table 3.
Alarm signs that favor organic diseases.

Condition	Diagnostic evaluation
Anatomic malformations of the colon and rectum	
Imperforate anus, anal or colonic stenosis, anteriorly displaced anus	Physical examination, barium enema
Spinal cord abnormalities	Spinal magnetic resonance imaging, anorectal manometry, urodynamics
Meningomyelocele, spinal cord tumor or trauma, tethered cord	
Metabolic conditions	
Hypothyroidism	Thyroid studies
Hypercalcemia, hyperkalemia	Serum calcium and potassium levels
Diabetes mellitus	Fasting glucose level
Diabetes insipidus	Serum and urine osmolarity
Neuropathic gastrointestinal disorders	
Hirschsprung's disease, internal anal sphincter achalasia	Anorectal manometry, rectal suction biopsy
Visceral myopathy/neuropathy	Colonic manometry
Drug use/toxin exposure	History, drug level
Opiates, phenobarbital, anticholinergics and attention-deficit/hyperactivity disorder drugs, antacids and sucralfate (Carafate), antidepressants, antihypertensives	Lead level
Lead toxicity	
Celiac disease	Sweat test
Cystic fibrosis	Cow's milk elimination
Cow's milk protein intolerance	Special testing
Connective tissue disorder, mitochondrial disorders	Psychological and psychiatric evaluation
Psychiatric disorders	
Functional constipation	History and physical examination; no testing

Table 4.
Differential diagnosis and evaluation of constipation in children.

be performed to exclude systemic diseases, such as hypothyroidism, celiac disease, or lead toxicity. Anorectal manometry can assess for sphincter abnormalities, such as Hirschsprung's disease or a nonrelaxing internal anal sphincter (IAS). Magnetic resonance imaging is uses to evaluate for a tethered cord, spinal cord tumor, or sacral agenesis [16, 17].

6. Treatment

6.1 Education and behavior modification/dietary changes

It is important to explain that overflow of stools leads to fecal pseudo-incontinence and is not an voluntary defiance. Regular toileting (for 5–10 min) after meals combined with a reward system is often helpful. Parents should expect gradual improvement with occasional relapses and encourage to maintain a positive and supportive attitude throughout the treatment. Although behavior modification may help in occasional cases, intensive behavior therapy does not seem to add to treatment success. Studies have shown that children with constipation have a lower fiber intake than other children. Too early and vigorous toilet training may be detrimental for the child. The child is encouraged to sit on the toilet for 5–10 min, 3–4 times a day immediately after major meals for initial months [11].

Dietary changes are often advised in children with constipation. Some authors suggest that increased intake of fluids and carbohydrates (e.g., sorbitol in prune, pear, and apple juice) can help soften stools, particularly in infants. A well-balanced diet that includes whole grains, fruits, and vegetables is recommended for children with constipation [12]. Guidelines do not support the following therapies for the treatment of childhood functional constipation: fiber supplements, extra fluid intake, routine use of pre- or probiotics, or alternative treatments such as acupuncturc or chiropractic therapy. Child with cow's milk intolerance may respond to a trial of a cow's milk-free diet, especially in young children with anal fissures [13].

6.2 Management of children with functional constipation

6.2.1 Initial treatment with disimpaction

Fecal impaction is diagnosed on per abdomen examination, digital rectal examination, or excessive stool in the colon identified by abdominal radiography. Disimpaction can either be performed by oral or rectal routes; studies have shown no significant differences between the two routes. Evidence shows that PEG and enemas are equally effective for fecal disimpaction. Polyethylene glycol is ideal for oral disimpaction at a dose of 1.5 g/kg/day for 3–6 days; maximum dose 100 g/day. Rectal disimpaction has also been effectively performed with glycerin suppositories in infants and bisacodyl suppositories in older children. Use of soap suds, tap water, and magnesium enemas is not recommended because of their potential toxicity [17].

6.2.2 Follow-up maintenance therapy

Lactulose is considered to be safe for all ages. Evidence shows that PEG is more effective compared with lactulose, milk of magnesia, mineral oil, or placebo.

Lactulose is recommended in case PEG is not available (JPGN). Some authors suggest medical therapy should be continued for at least the time since a child had constipation. Regular follow-up (by reviewing stool records and repeating abdominal and (if required) rectal examination) is a key to the success of functional constipation. As mentioned above, dosage adjustment may be needed. Once a regular bowel habit is established, the laxative dosage is to be decreased gradually before stopping [18]. Parents should maintain a daily record (stool diary) of bowel movements, fecal soiling, pain or discomfort, consistency of stool, and the laxative dose. This helps in modification of dosage of laxatives (**Table 5**). About 50% will recover, and will be without laxatives after 6–12 months. Approximately, an additional 10% is well while taking laxatives, and 40% will still be symptomatic despite the use of laxatives. Children with early age of presentation (<4 years), associated with fecal incontinence, and history of longer duration of symptoms (>6 months) have poor outcome [3].

6.2.3 Refractory constipation

Refractory constipation is defined when there is no response to optimal conventional treatment for at least 3 months. The refractory constipation has a prevalence of 20–30%, but the prevalence is much higher in underdeveloped countries like India [19]. While managing a case of refractory constipation common organic causes (Hirschsprung disease, hypothyroidism, celiac disease, hypercalcemia, spinal cord abnormalities) should be ruled out first. Motility studies like colon transit time (CTT), anorectal manometry with balloon expulsion test, and colonic manometry should be performed to rule out organic causes before labelling constipation as refractory [20].

6.2.4 Slow transient constipation

In radiographic CTT study, after oral administration of radio-opaque markers, radiograph of abdomen is taken sequentially on the fourth and seventh day; X-ray markers are counted in right colon; and if retention of contrast occurs after 62 h, it is called as slow transient constipation. Clinical features of slow transit constipation in these children include history of delayed passage of meconium, onset of symptoms early of symptoms early in first year and/or failure to toilet training, feces soft rather than rock hard, high fiber diets worsen the symptoms, and delay in colonic transit on transit study [21]. The management of slow transit constipation is challenging as they do not respond to conventional laxative therapy and the main concern is soiling. Fiber therapy is contraindicated. The only effective therapy for this subset of patients is antegrade continence enema. Malone antegrade continence enema (MACE) helps in refractory slow transit constipation cases [22]. Appendix is exteriorized as small

Drugs	Dose	Side effects
Lactulose	1–2 g/kg, 1–2 doses	Bloating, abdominal cramps
Milk of magnesia	1–3 mL/kg/day, 1–2 doses	Hypocalcemia, hypermagnesemia, hypophosphatemia
PEG for disimpaction	25 mL/kg/h (R/T) or 1–1.5 g/kg	Nausea, bloating, cramps, vomiting
PEG for maintenance	5–10 mL/kg/day or 0.4–0.8 g/kg/	Nausea, bloating, cramps, vomiting
Bisacodyl	0.5–1 suppository (10 mg) 1–3 tabs/dose	Abdominal pain, diarrhea, hypokalemia
Senna	2–6 years: 2.5–7.5 mL/day (8.8 mg/5 mL)	Melanosis coli, hepatitis, hypertrophic 6–12 years: 5–15 mL/day osteoarthropathy, neuropathy

Table 5.
Laxatives-dosage and side effects.

opening on to the skin. Colonic manometry results should be optimal before contemplating MACE.

Internal anal sphincter achalasia (IAS) is a rare but important cause of refractory constipation. In a study of 332 patients with severe constipation, De Caluwe et al. [23] have reported this as a cause in just 4.5% of cases. This is associated with severe constipation and incontinence. It is diagnosed by the absence of anorectal inhibitory reflex (ARIR) on anorectal manometry along with the presence of ganglion cell on rectal. Sphincter myectomy is more rewarding than intrasphincteric botulinum toxin injection.

7. Conclusions

Functional constipation is quite common in both developed and not developed nations and is benign. Parent education, toilet training, dietary changes, initial moral or rectal disimpaction and use of appropriate laxative and follow-up of the responses to the treatment are keystone of successful management. Meticulous history and proper physical examination, including digital rectal examination, can differentiate functional from organic constipation. Treatment in functional constipation can be started before any investigation. Disimpaction either with oral polyethylene glycol or rectal enemas is the first step in the management of constipation. Polyethylene glycol is more effective but costlier than lactulose. At times, prolonged maintenance of laxative therapy (months to years) may be required and noncompliance leads to recurrence. Radiological colon transit time is useful in the management of refractory constipation. Slow transit constipation is a different entity, and Malone continence enema helps in this subset of patients. Some pathological and surgical causes need to be ruled out if warning signs or symptoms are present, which may require contrast enema, anorectal manometry, and rectal biopsy.

Author details

Raashid Hamid* and Shazada Shahid Banday
Department of Pediatric and Neonatal Surgery, Sheri-I-Kashmir Institute of Medical Sciences, Soura, Srinagar, Jammu and Kashmir, India

*Address all correspondence to: drraashidhamid@gmail.com

References

[1] Benninga M, Candy DC, Catto-Smith AG, et al. The Paris Consensus on Childhood Constipation Terminology (PACCT) Group. Journal of Pediatric Gastroenterology and Nutrition. 2005;**40**:273-275

[2] Weaver LT, Steiner H. The bowel habits of young children. Archives of Disease in Childhood. 1983;**59**:649-652

[3] Poddar U. Approach to constipation in children. Indian Pediatrics. 2016;**53**:319-327

[4] Southwell BR, Clarke MC, Sutcliffe J, et al. Colonic transit studies: Normal values for adults and children with comparison of radiological and scintigraphic methods. Pediatric Surgery International. 2009;**25**:559-572

[5] Hyman PE, Milla PJ, Benninga MA, Davidson GP, Fleisher DF, Taminiau J. Childhood functional gastrointestinal disorders: Neonate/toddler. Gastroenterology. 2006;**130**:1519-1526

[6] Baucke VL. Prevalence, symptoms and outcome of constipation in infants and toddlers. The Journal of Pediatrics. 2005;**146**:359-363

[7] Loening-Baucke V. Chronic constipation in children. Gastroenterology. 1993;**105**:1557-1564

[8] Loening-Baucke V. Constipation in early childhood: Patient characteristics, treatment and long-term followup. Gut. 1993;**34**:1400-1404

[9] Kehar M, Yadav SP, Sachdeva A. Constipation in children. JIMSA. 2012;**25**:31-33

[10] Khanna V, Poddar U, Yachha SK. Constipation in Indian children: Need for knowledge not the knife. Indian Pediatrics. 2010;**47**:1025-1030

[11] Loening-Baucke V. Polyethylene glycol without electrolytes for children with constipation and encopresis. Journal of Pediatric Gastroenterology and Nutrition. 2002;**34**:372-377

[12] Benninga MA, Buller HA, Staalman CR, Gubler FM, Bossuyt PM, van der Plas RN, et al. Defecation disorders in children, colonic transit times versus the Barr-score. European Journal of Pediatrics. 1995;**154**:277-284

[13] Tabbers MM, Di Lorenzo C, Berger MY, Faure C, Langendam MW, Nurko S, et al. Evaluation and treatment of functional constipation in infants and children: Evidence-based recommendations from ESPGHAN and NASPGHAN. Journal of Pediatric Gastroenterology and Nutrition. 2014;**58**:25874

[14] Taitz LS, Water JKH, Urwin OM, Molnar D. Factors associated with outcome in management of defecation disorders. Archives of Disease in Childhood. 1986;**61**:472-477

[15] Partin JC, Hamill SK, Fischel JE, Partin JS. Painful defecation and fecal soiling in children. Pediatrics. 1992;**89**:1007-1009

[16] Metaj M, Laroia N, Lawrence RA, Ryan RM. Comparison of breast- and formula-fed normal new born in time to first stool and urine. Journal of Perinatology. 2003;**23**:624-628

[17] Jung PM. Hirschsprung's disease: One surgeon's experience in one institution. Journal of Pediatric Surgery. 1995;**30**:646-651

[18] Candy D, Belsey J. Macrogol (polyethylene glycol) laxatives in children with functional constipation and fecal impaction: A systematic review. Archives of Disease in Childhood. 2009;**94**:156-160

[19] Southwell BR, King SK, Hutson JM. Chronic constipation in children: Organic disorders are a major cause. Journal of Paediatrics and Child Health. 2005;**41**:1-15

[20] Kwshtgar A, Ward HC, Clayden GS. Diagnosis and management of children with intractable constipation. Seminars in Pediatric Surgery. 2004;**13**:300-309

[21] Hutson JM, McNamara J, Gibb S, Shin YM. Slow transit constipation in children. Journal of Paediatrics and Child Health. 2001;**37**:426-430

[22] Malone PS, Ransley PG, Kiely EM. Preliminary report: The antegrade continence enema. Lancet. 1990;**336**:1217-1218

[23] De Caluwe D, Yoneda A, Akl U, Puri P. Internal anal sphincter achalasia: Outcome after internal sphincter myectomy. Journal of Pediatric Surgery. 2001;**36**:736-738

Chapter 3

Prevalence and Treatment of Constipation in Patients with Alpha-Synuclein Pathology

Charles M. Lepkowsky

Abstract

α-Synuclein "Lewy body" pathology is the basis of Parkinson's disease (PD) and neurocognitive disorder with Lewy bodies (NCDLB), sometimes called Lewy body dementia. In patients with α-synuclein pathology, constipation, obstipation and impaction are almost universal symptoms, whose treatment represents a significant burden on health care economies. Description is given of the specific mechanisms through which α-synuclein pathology induces these symptoms, and through which the use of acetylcholinesterase inhibitors (AChEIs) might significantly reduce them. Four case studies are presented testing the hypothesis that the use of the cholinergic agonist donepezil might reduce the symptom of constipation in four patients with NCDLB or PD at different stages of disease progression. Outcomes are presented, as well as follow-up data at 6-, 12-, and 18-month intervals. The potential use of donepezil to reduce the symptoms of constipation in patients with α-synuclein pathology is discussed.

Keywords: constipation, α-Synuclein pathology, Parkinson's disease, neurocognitive disorder with Lewy bodies, Lewy body dementia, acetylcholinesterase inhibitors (AChEIs)

1. Introduction

Longevity has increased significantly over the past four decades [1], bringing with it a significant increase in the number of older adults affected by neurocognitive diseases (formerly called dementias) [2]. Worldwide, the number of people diagnosed with neurocognitive disease was 46.8 million in 2015, and 50 million in 2017. This figure is expected to exceed 75 million by 2030, and 131.5 million by 2050 [3–5]. Approximately 67% of dementia diagnoses are assigned to Alzheimer's disease (AD), 22% to neurocognitive disorder with Lewy bodies (NCDLB) (previously called Lewy body dementia), and the remaining 9% to Parkinson's disease (PD) [2].

According to the US Census Bureau, the Center for Medicare and Medicaid Services (CMS) and the U.S. Burden of Disease Collaborators, the largest increases in annual payments for treatment and long-term care for older adults were for those diagnosed with neurocognitive disease. Per capita, PD and NCDLB represent more than their numeric percentage of this expense, which grew 113 percent between 1990 and 2010. Worldwide in 2015, the estimated economic burden of

AD	Alzheimer's Disease
PD	Parkinson's Disease
NCDLB	Neurocognitive disorder with Lewy Bodies
CNS	Central nervous system
ANS	Autonomic nervous system
PNS	Peripheral nervous system
ENS	Enteric nervous system
MCI	Mild cognitive impairment
ACh	Acetlycholine
AChE	Acetylcholinesterase
AChEI	Acetylcholinesterase inhibitor
REM	Rapid eye movement
RBD	REM behavior disorder
RSWA	REM sleep without dystonia
MP	Myenteric plexus
SMCP	Submucosal colonic plexus
ER	Endoplasmic reticulum
MMSE	Mini mental status exam
QDRS	Quick dementia rating system
LBCRS	Lewy body composite risk score
OTC	Over the counter
HS	Taken daily
PRN	As needed
MRI	Magnetic resonance imaging
CMS	Center for medicare and medicaid services
APA	American Psychological Association

Table 1.
Abbreviations.

neurocognitive disease was $818 billion, representing 1.09% of global gross domestic product. Currently, the global cost of neurocognitive disease is estimated above $1 trillion, and is expected to increase fourfold to more than $4 trillion by 2050 [2, 6, 7]. As the occurrence of neurocognitive disease increases, early and accurate diagnosis becomes increasingly important for appropriate treatment, as well as containment of the cost associated with care delivery.

So what are PD and NCDLB, and why do they cost so much to treat?

PD and NCDLB are α-synuclein "Lewy body "pathologies characterized by a wide range of cognitive, motor, and autonomic symptoms, including constipation, obstipation, and impaction [8]. The disproportionate cost of care for α-synucleopathologies is due to their widely varied symptom presentation, combined with significant, progressive debilitation within systems affected by Lewy bodies. Lewy bodies are abnormal intracellular aggregations of α-synuclein protein [9]. α-synuclein pathology, α-synucleopathology, and α-synucleinopathy are all terms used to describe impairment of neural functioning due to the presence of Lewy Bodies (aggregates of α-synuclein protein) [10].

Pertinent to the topic of constipation, escalating gastric immotility in PD and NCDLB compromises mobility, sleep, cognition, and mood, increasing the cost of care, and potentially debilitating and/or dramatically reducing the quality of life for patients [11–17]. Although gastric immotility is a prevalent symptom characteristic of α-synuclein disorders, constipation, obstipation, and impaction are rarely a focus of treatment for patients with PD and NCDLB [18]. When PD and NCDLB constipation, obstipation, and impaction are addressed, primary care physicians typically recommend conventional (often over-the-counter) treatments, despite data demonstrating that such treatments are ineffective with this population [12]. In order to make accurate diagnosis and assign appropriate and effective treatment, it is necessary to understand constipation, obstipation, and impaction as symptomatic manifestations of Lewy (α-synuclein) pathology in the enteric nervous system (ENS), and the specific mechanisms through which synuclein pathology impairs bowel motility. Medical intervention can then be selected based on the use of medications known to counteract those mechanisms. The effectiveness of evidence-based medical intervention can be evaluated through large data set studies, and/or longitudinal case studies.

In this chapter, Lewy pathology in PD and NCDLB and its symptomatic manifestations in the ENS will be described. The specific mechanisms through which α-synucleopathology causes those symptoms will be explained, followed by a description of the mechanisms though which specific medications counter those of α-synuclein proteins. A series of case studies will be described, in which four patients at different stages of disease progression with NCDLB or PD were each treated using medication with demonstrated effectiveness for countering the mechanisms underlying α-synucleinopathy in the ENS. Outcomes will be reviewed at 6, 12, and 18 month follow-up intervals, followed by a discussion of implications for future research and practice. Abbreviations used in this chapter are summarized in **Table 1**.

2. α-Synuclein pathology: Lewy bodies in PD and NCDLB

Unlike Alzheimer's disease (AD), which is associated with presence of two proteins in the central nervous system (CNS), amyloid-β (Aβ) and tau, PD and NCDLB are diseases characterized by the presence of Lewy bodies, pathologic aggregates of the synaptic protein α-synuclein. In PD and NCDLB, Lewy bodies appear not only in the CNS, but also in the autonomic nervous system (ANS), the peripheral nervous system (PNS) and the enteric nervous system (ENS), spreading from one nervous system area to the next over time [19, 20]. In PD and NCDLB patients, there is evidence that Lewy bodies travel from the gut to the brain, or vice-versa [21, 22]. Lewy bodies aggregate not only near the nucleus of the neuron, but even more abundantly in neurites (axons and dendrites) [23].

2.1 Symptomatic manifestations of α-synuclein pathology

While amyloid-β (Aβ) and tau pathology in AD are associated almost exclusively with cognitive impairment in the CNS, Lewy pathology in PD and NCDLB is heterogeneous in its presentation. Not every PD or NCDLB patient has the same, or all, α-synuclein pathology symptoms.

Most Lewy body patients present with disordered sleep: REM Sleep Behavior Disorder (RBD), and especially REM sleep without atonia (RSWA). They act out their dreams, sometimes injuring their bed partner, or remaining sleepless at night and drowsy all day [24]. Many Lewy body patients present with ANS dysfunction, including urinary incontinence, constipation, erectile dysfunction, coronary dysfunction, or orthostatic hypotension, which increases the likelihood of injury due to falling [25, 26]. Lewy body patients sometimes present with sensory dysfunction, losing their sense of smell (anosmia) [27], and/or seeing colors differently [28]. Some Lewy body patients initially present with late life onset depression, with or without visual or auditory hallucinations, delusions, and anxiety [29]. Lewy body patients sometimes initially present with cognitive impairment, including attentional deficits, short-term memory loss, and/or difficulty with concentration or word-finding. Most often these symptoms are functionally diagnosed as Mild Cognitive Impairment (MCI), and frequently, later in symptom progression as AD, which is a common misdiagnosis [30]. Lewy body patients presenting with evolving Parkinsonian features (including shuffling gait, weakness, pain in muscles and joints, and/or tremor) are most often diagnosed with PD, which might be correct, or might be a misdiagnosis overlooking or minimizing the relevance of other symptoms listed above [31]. In some Lewy body patients, Parkinsonian features might not appear at all, or until long after other symptoms have become more prevalent [32].

Constellations of three or more of these symptom presentations are considered reliable prodromal indicators of α-synucleopathology, as well as differential diagnostic indicators distinguishing NCDLB from AD [8]. Proper identification of prodromal Lewy body symptoms for early and accurate diagnosis of α-synucleopathology reduces the likelihood of misdiagnosis, and facilitates early treatment intervention to minimize or delay the emergence of multi-nervous system symptoms that impair functioning and reduce quality of life, with the consequent benefit of containing the cost of care delivery. Early diagnosis has been hindered more by general unawareness of prodromal symptom constellations with demonstrated predictive accuracy for α-synucleopathology [8] than by an actual lack of reliable biomarkers for α-synucleopathology [33].

Although Lewy body patients demonstrate wide variation in symptom presentation, the symptom almost universal to patients diagnosed with PD and NCDLB is constipation, which can lead to obstipation and/or impaction [14, 26, 34–44]. The uniformity of gastric immotility in patients with PD and NCDLB suggests that α-synuclein pathology directly affects the enteric nervous system (ENS).

2.2 Symptomatic manifestations of α-synuclein pathology in the ENS

Because gastric immotility is such a consistent symptom feature of PD and NCDLB, much research has focused on whether or to what extent Lewy pathology occurs in the ENS of PD & NCDLB patients. Research data consistently demonstrate that abnormal α-synuclein proteins aggregate in the ENS of patients diagnosed with PD and NCDLB, with symptomatic manifestation as gastric immotility [14, 26, 34–44]. In patients diagnosed with PD, symptoms frequently include increased colonic transit time [45] and impaired gastric emptying [46]. In PD patients, constipation is at least three times as prevalent as it is among the general population [47], and several researchers believe that constipation is a universal feature of PD [48]. In both PD and NCDLB, the symptom of bowel immotility often presents years before other diagnostic features [47, 49–53] sometimes as much as 20 years before the emergence of others symptoms leading to the diagnosis of PD or NCDLB [17]. This occurs so frequently that many experts suggest that bowel immotility is a prodromal symptom for both PD and NCDLB [17, 21, 25, 37, 54–57].

3. The mechanism of α-synuclein impairment of the ENS

In patients with PD and NCDLB, high concentrations Lewy bodies (α-synuclein protein aggregates) are found in the myenteric plexus (MP) [56, 58–63] and the colonic submucosal plexus (CSMP) [40]. 95% of innervation in the MP and the CSMP is cholinergic, and the CSMP is innervated by the MP [64]. As in other neurotransmitter pathways, Lewy bodies in the MP and CSMP do not appear exclusively in the form of large aggregations of α-synuclein protein near the nucleus. Small aggregations of α-synuclein and other proteins aggregate even more abundantly in neurites (axons and dendrites) [65]. The abundance of Lewy bodies in the predominantly cholinergic neurotransmitter pathways innervating the MP and CSMP interferes with cholinergic neurotransmission.

The specific biochemical mechanisms posited for α-synuclein pathology-based reduction of cholinergic functioning include endoplasmic reticulum (ER) stress, blockage in endoplasmic reticulum (ER)-to-Golgi vesicular trafficking, and mitochondrial dysfunction, all of which contribute to α-synuclein-induced cell death [66–68]. The degeneration of cholinergic neurons leads to a decline in levels of acetylcholine (ACh) [69]. The loss of cholinergic function in the MP and the CSMP reduces or eliminates signals that induce and maintain peristalsis, symptomatically manifesting as constipation, obstipation, and/or impaction [8, 13, 17, 23, 44, 46, 52, 70–73]. The presence of Lew bodies in the MP and CSMP predates cognitive and motor functional manifestations of α-synuclein diseases [42, 61] so consistently that it has been nominated as a potential biomarker for α-synuclein pathology [74].

3.1 Potential exacerbation of ENS symptoms by anti-Parkinson medication

In both PD and NCDLB, α-synuclein patients with Parkinsonian features are often prescribed L-dopa agents such as carbidopa-levodopa (known also by the brand names Sinemet and Stalevo) in order to preserve gait, balance, and other basic motor functions [18, 75, 76]. Complicating or exacerbating gastric immotility due to α-synuclein ENS pathology, carbidopa-levodopa's potential side effects include constipation [77]. Other medications frequently used to mitigate resting tremor in PD and NCDLB include trihexyphenidyl (marketed as Artane or Trihex) and benztropine mesylate (marketed as Cogentin). Each has been identified as an anticholinergic medication, which accordingly can also exacerbate gastric immotility through suppression of the cholinergic neurotransmitter pathways innervating the ENS [76, 78–80].

4. The mechanism of symptom relief for cholinergic α-synuclein pathology: cholinergic agonist use in NCDLB and PD

The symptomatic features of PD and NCDLB have long been known to include cholinergic neural deficits and functional impairment [81–87]. Over time, it has become increasingly evident that α-synuclein pathology is the basis of cholinergic impairments in PD and NCDLB [82, 87, 88].[1] With the hope of mitigating α-synuclein cholinergic impairment [29, 65, 88, 91, 92], cholinergic agonists such as acetylcholinesterase inhibitors (AChEIs) are prescribed to NCDLB and PD patients. AChEIs include tacrine, galantamine, rivastigmine, and donepezil.

Low doses of tacrine have been associated with reductions of motor symptoms in PD patients [80] and galantamine [93]. Rivastigmine has been used to reduce neuropsychiatric symptoms and improve cognitive function as measured by the

[1] Cholinergic impairment does not appear to be a consistent finding in Alzheimer's disease (AD) [86, 91]. Research consistently demonstrates that autonomic dysfunction is a feature of PD and NCDLB, but not AD [25, 39, 82, 89], and that alpha-synuclein expression is increased in NCDLB and PD, but not in AD [35, 41, 90]. For this reason, AD is not included in this discussion.

Mini-Mental State Exam (MMSE) [94] in patients with NCDLB [95–98]. In PD patients, however, the use of Rivastigmine to improve cognition has also been associated with higher rates of nausea, vomiting, and tremor [99].[2]

Donepezil has been used to improve cognition and reduce hallucinations and delusions in PD patients with cognitive impairment (suggesting that they are in fact NCDLB patients) [107]. 5–10 mg daily dosages of donepezil used in conjunction with antiparkinsonian therapy produced significant reduction in psychotic symptoms in PD patients (again, likely misdiagnosed NCDLB patients), without apparent side effects or exacerbation of Parkinsonian symptoms [108]. An early study suggested that treatment of NCDLB with donepezil was sometimes associated with an increase in Parkinsonian features [109]. However, a large body of subsequent research indicates that donepezil reduces neurocognitive symptoms in patients with NCDLB without worsening Parkinsonian features [110–120], and a Cochrane database systematic review of previous research using cholinergic agonists to treat PD & NCDLB found that donepezil produced consistent reduction in neurocognitive symptoms without exacerbation of Parkinsonian features or other side effects [121].

When compared to other acetylcholinesterase inhibitors including Galantamine and Rivastigmine for use with patients diagnosed with PD and NCDLB, donepezil has performed well, improving cognition [122], but with fewer side effects [123]. PD and NCDLB patients treated with donepezil demonstrated significant improvements in cognition and behavior which disappeared when donepezil was withdrawn, and later showed restoration of treatment gains upon recommencement of donepezil [124]. In patients with NCDLB, long-term administration of donepezil at 10 mg/day has been shown to improve cognitive function for up to 52 weeks without increasing the risk of Parkinsonian features or other clinically significant safety events [125, 126].

4.1 Donepezil for symptom relief of constipation

Conventional treatments for constipation have proven ineffective in older patients in residential settings, especially for patients with neurocognitive disorders [12]. Recalling that 95% of the innervation of the MP and CSMP in the ENS is cholinergic [64], it is interesting to note that donepezil has been shown to reduce ANS symptoms including constipation in nongeriatric affective patients [127]. Donepezil increases cholinergically mediated bowel contractions as much as 477% in patients suffering from severe intestinal dysmotility [128]. The mechanisms through which donepezil mitigates these symptoms is twofold. AChEIs like donepezil inhibit the action of the ACh-hydrolyzing enzyme acetylcholinesterase (AChE), increasing ACh levels, with consequent reduction in symptoms associated with progressive cholinergic dysfunction [69]. Donepezil is a specific, reversible AChE inhibitor [129, 130]. Donepezil also interacts independently with neuronal nicotinic ACh receptors [131]. Donepezil's dual action has made it a long-standing choice for countering cholinergic impairment [69, 124, 131].

4.2 A hypothetical model for symptom relief of cholinergic α-synuclein pathology in the ENS

On the basis of substantial research a) linking constipation in patients with NCDLB and PD to α-synucleopathology-based impairment of cholinergic function in the MP and CSMP in the ENS, b) demonstrating that the use of the donepezil as

[2] Rare, potentially dangerous side effects of cholinergic agonists include rhabdomyolysis and neuroleptic malignant syndrome (NMS) [100–106].

a cholinergic agonist mitigates cholinergic impairment in α-synuclein pathology patients, and c) showing that the use of the donepezil increases bowel motility in non-geriatric patients with gastric immotility, it was postulated that the use of donepezil might counter α-synuclein pathological impairment of the MP and CSMP in patients with NCDLB and PD, leading to increased bowel motility and a consequent reduction in the symptom of constipation.

PD patients and NCDLB patients with significant Parkinsonian features are frequently prescribed L-dopa agents like carbidopa-levodopa (known also by the brand name Sinemet) to preserve balance, gait, and other basic motor functions [31, 76]. Carbidopa-Levodopa's potential side effects include constipation [77]. Accordingly, it was postulated that the use of donepezil might have specific benefit in reducing constipation in patients with PD and NCDLB receiving L-dopa agents like carbidopa-levodopa.

To test these hypotheses, in a series of case studies donepezil was prescribed to four PD and NCDLB patients at different stages of disease progression, each suffering from constipation, obstipation, and/or impaction. Discussion of other diagnoses, symptoms, or treatments is limited, in order to make the case studies as brief as possible, while maintaining focus on donepezil's potential for reducing constipation, obstipation, and impaction.

5. Four case studies: methods

5.1 Case study #1

Mr. A. was a non-Hispanic white male 50–55 years of age. He had been diagnosed with PD. His presenting symptoms included depression, transient hand tremor, cognitive interference resulting in permanent disability work status, lower back pain, insomnia, and significant constipation, with frequency of bowel movements about once a week. For treatment of his Parkinsonian symptoms, the patient had been treated for 2 years with carbidopa-levodopa (Sinemet) and pramipexole (Mirapex) (both dopamine agonists). He had also been prescribed acetaminophen/oxycodone (Percoset) for back pain, and dronabinol (Marinol) for pain and insomnia. For constipation, he had been advised to use over the counter (OTC) products including stewed prunes, prune juice, psyllium (fiber), and Senokot laxative/stool softener. None of the OTC remedies had produced any reduction in the symptom of constipation.

Donepezil was prescribed at a starting dose of 5 mg per day. Within 2 weeks, the patient reported that his frequency of bowel movements had increased to every other day. After 4 weeks, the frequency of bowel movements had increased to once a day. There was no increase in Parkinsonian features or other clinically significant symptoms, nor was there emergence of new symptoms.

5.2 Case study #2

Ms. B. was a non-Hispanic white female 65–70 years of age. She had not yet received a neurocognitive or Parkinsonian diagnosis, but had been diagnosed with late-life onset of acute anxiety and depression without suicidal ideation, in addition to standing diagnoses of hypertension, hypothyroid, and possible sleep apnea. For several years she had received prescriptive Spironolactone 25 mg HS (as a diuretic), Levothyroxine 75 mcg HS (for hypothyroid), and most recently Lorazepam 1 mg PRN (for anxiety). Her presenting symptoms included cognitive interference (short-term memory loss and difficulty word-finding), agitation, panic attacks, dysphoria, insomnia (onset, median, and terminal waking), restless sleep (which her spouse described as talking and flailing in her sleep), and constipation (of approximately 5 years). At intake, the patient reported that the frequency of bowel movements was approximately twice a week. She had tried a variety of OTC and dietary remedies, all of which had been ineffective. The patient was administered the MMSE [94], the Quick Dementia Rating Scale (QDRS) [132] and the Lewy Body Composite Risk Score (LBCRS) [133]. Her scores indicated mild cognitive impairment (MCI) and suggested neurocognitive impairment consistent with that found in patients with Lewy body disorders. In combination, the symptoms of MCI, late-life onset depression, and sleep disturbance (possible REM sleep behavior disorder or RSBD and/or REM sleep without atonia, or RSWA) [105] are considered prodromal for NCDLB. A neurological evaluation and a sleep study were ordered in order to gather confirmatory evidence. The neurological assessment confirmed MCI, and an MRI showed reduced cerebral (white matter) volume. RSBD/RSWA was confirmed by the sleep study.

Donepezil was prescribed at a starting dose of 5 mg per day. Within 3 weeks the patient reported that her frequency of bowel movements had increased to about every other day. After 5 weeks, she reported daily bowel movements. There was no exacerbation of Parkinsonian features or other clinically significant symptoms.

5.3 Case study #3

Mr. C. was a non-Hispanic white male 65–70 years of age recently diagnosed with Major Depressive Disorder, with history of cervical vertebral fusions C5–C7. His presenting symptoms included cognitive interference (short-term memory loss and difficulty word-finding), panic attacks, appetite suppression, generalized anxiety, frequent migraine headaches, feeling off balance, dysphoria, insomnia (onset, median and terminal waking), restless sleep (which his spouse described as yelling and striking out in his sleep), and constipation (for about 4 years). OTC and dietary treatments had not been effective for reducing the symptom of constipation. To treat his anxiety and depression, the patient had recently been prescribed Paroxetine HCl (Paxil) 30 mg daily, and for his panic and anxiety, clonazepam (Klonopin) 0.5 mg PRN. The patient was administered the MMSE, the QDRS and the LBCRS. His scores indicated mild cognitive impairment (MCI) and suggested neurocognitive impairment consistent with that found in patients with Lewy body disorders. The patient soon began to complain of increasing difficulties with balance, gait, and weakness. His depression increased, and he began to report suicidal ideation. He stated that his appetite suppression and constipation had both increased. During the same time frame, the patient's cognitive impairment escalated rapidly. The combination of symptoms including MCI, rapid cognitive changes, balance/gait impairment, late-life onset depression and anxiety, weakness, appetite suppression, constipation, and sleep disturbance (possible REM sleep behavior disorder or RSBD and/or REM sleep without atonia, or RSWA) is consistent with the diagnosis of NCDLB. A neurological evaluation and a sleep study were ordered. Although an MRI was unrevealing, the neurological assessment was confirmatory for MCI. The sleep study confirmed the diagnosis of RSBD/RSWA.

Paroxetine is known to have anticholinergic properties [134], so its use was discontinued. Sertraline 100 mg per day was prescribed, and within weeks was increased to 200 mg per day. The PRN dosage of Clonazepam was increased to 0.75 mg. Abilify (aripiprazole) 1 mg per day was added to address the patient's intractable depression. Topiramate 75 mg HS was prescribed for the migraine headaches. To address the sleep disturbance, melatonin 6 mg and Mirtazapine 30 mg were prescribed for use at bedtime. It was hoped that mirtazapine might potentiate the effects of the Sertraline, while reducing restlessness in bed. The patient reported reductions in depression. However, there appeared to be no reduction in RSBD/RSWA. To address the patient's rapidly advancing cognitive impairment, Memantine was prescribed 10 mg morning and at night, which produced significant cognitive improvement. To address the balance issues, tremor, gait disturbance, and general weakness, carbidopa-levodopa (Sinemet) 25/100 mg was prescribed three times a day, soon producing improvement in motor function. However, during the same time period, the symptom of constipation intensified. The patient reported that the frequency of bowel movements had fallen to less than once per week. OTC and dietary remedies had not produced any improvement. During this time frame, the patient became impacted twice, and each time had to be treated in the emergency room using bowel voiding medications intended for colonoscopies or bowel surgical procedures.

Donepezil was prescribed at a starting dose of 2.5 mg per day. The patient reported that during the first 2 weeks, his bowel movement frequency had increased to once every other day. After 4 weeks, he reported that the frequency of his bowel movements had increased to once a day. There was no change in the frequency of bowel movements for the next 3 months, but the patient expressed concern that his appetite and bowel production were not adequate. In an effort to achieve further symptom improvement, the dosage of donepezil was increased to 5 mg per day. Within days, there were improvements in appetite, volume of dietary intake, and bowel output. There was no increase in Parkinsonian features or other clinically significant symptoms.

Following the increase in donepezil to 5 mg daily, the patient and his spouse described significant improvement in his cognitive functioning, including word finding and short-term memory. The patient was again administered the MMSE, the QDRS and the LBCRS. His scores had improved significantly on all three instruments, suggesting overall recovery of cognitive function.

5.4 Case study #4

Mr. D. was a non-Hispanic white male 75–80 years of age. He had recently been diagnosed with PD and Major Depressive Disorder, with history of hypercholesterolemia, arteriosclerosis, lower back surgery, coronary artery stent replacement, small bowel obstruction, peripheral vascular disease, and chronic lower back pain. His presenting symptoms included cognitive interference (short-term memory loss and difficulty with word-finding), generalized anxiety, blunted affect, appetite suppression, depression, passive suicidal ideation, lower back pain, weakness, hand tremor, motor retardation, difficulties with balance, tottering or shuffling gait, sleep disturbance (onset, median and terminal waking), and constipation. At intake, he reported the frequency of bowel movements at approximately twice a week. OTC and dietary treatments had not been effective in reducing his constipation. The patient stated that for several years, he had experienced difficulties with balance. He sought referral to an orthopedist, and ultimately underwent surgery. The patient reported that subsequent to the surgery, he experienced chronic lower back pain, which was significant enough to interfere with routine activities. He ceased routine physical exercise, reported increasing weakness over the past few months, lost confidence in his coordination, leading him to give up driving, and stated that his hand tremor had evolved to the extent that his handwriting was no longer legible. He described a deepening depression and the emergence of suicidal ideation. There was no report or evidence of symptoms consistent with RSBD or RSWA. However, the patient reported that the his constipation had increased and remained unresponsive to OTC or dietary remedies.

The patient was administered the MMSE, the QDRS and the LBCRS. His scores suggested mild cognitive impairment (MCI) and neurocognitive impairment consistent with that found in patients with Lewy body disorders. The combination of symptoms including cognitive impairment, blunt affect, anxiety, late-life onset depression, motor retardation, hand tremor, handwriting changes, lower back pain, weakness, impaired/shuffling gait, difficulties with balance, sleep disturbance, appetite suppression, and constipation is consistent with the diagnosis of NCDLB. A neurological evaluation and a sleep study were ordered. The neurological assessment confirmed the diagnosis of MCI, and an MRI indicated reduced cerebral (white matter) volume. The sleep study confirmed the diagnosis of RSBD/RSWA.

Donepezil was prescribed at a starting dosage of 5 mg per day. After 2 weeks, the patient reported that the frequency of his bowel movements had increased to about every other day. Within 3 weeks, he reported that he was having bowel movements every day. He also reported that his appetite had significantly increased. There was no exacerbation of Parkinsonian features or other clinically significant symptoms.

6. Results

6.1 Case study initial results

In each of the four patients in the case studies, the use of donepezil significantly reduced the symptom of constipation within a few weeks, without increasing Parkinsonian features or other clinically significant symptoms. There was also significant reduction of constipation for each of the two patients prescribed carbidopa-levodopa. In addition, when the patient whose NCDLB symptom progression was most advanced was readministered the MMSE, the QDRS and the LBCRS, he scored higher on all three tests, indicating improvements in overall cognitive functioning, word finding, and short-term memory.

6.2 Case study six-month follow-up

The symptom status of the four patients was reviewed 6 months later. The two patients in case studies #1 and #2 showed no symptom change. The two patients in case studies #3 and #4 each showed evidence of Lewy body symptom progression, including increased cognitive interference (short-term memory loss and difficulty with word-finding), generalized anxiety, dysphoric mood, blunted affect, appetite suppression, passive suicidal ideation, sleep disturbance (onset, median and terminal waking, REM sleep behavior disorder or RSBD and/or REM sleep without atonia, or RSWA), and Parkinsonian features (motor retardation, joint and muscle pain, reduced range of motion, diminished strength and coordination, increased tremor, gait disturbances, and difficulties with balance). Constipation, however, had not increased for any of the patients, nor was there evidence of new symptom emergence. Coincident with the 6 month symptom review, the patient in case study #3 had his dosage of donepezil doubled, from 5 to 10 mg orally administered daily, with the intention of mitigating his neurocognitive symptom progression.

6.3 Case study twelve-month follow-up

Twelve months after the initial findings had been reported, the symptom status of the four patients was again reviewed. During the interval between the 6 month and 12 month reviews, there was no apparent progression of Lewy body symptoms in any of the four patients. At 6 months, the patient in case study #3 had his dosage of donepezil doubled (from 5 to 10 mg orally administered daily) to address the progression of neurocognitive symptoms. At 12 months, he demonstrated reduced cognitive interference (short-term memory loss and difficulty with word-finding), which appeared to be associated with the increase in his dosage of donepezil. No other symptom changes were evident in that patient. In the remaining three patients, no symptom progression or change was apparent. None of the patients exhibited new symptoms, or any increase in the symptoms of constipation, obstipation, or impaction.

6.4 Case study eighteen-month follow-up

At 18 months, the symptom status of each of the four patients in the case studies was again reviewed. There was no apparent progression of Lewy body symptoms in any of the four patients between the 12 month and 18 month reviews. In the patient in case study #3, whose Lewy body symptoms had progressed at 6 months, doubling the dosage of donepezil (from 5 to 10 mg orally administered daily) continued to be associated with reduced cognitive interference (short-term memory loss and difficulty with word-finding). No other symptom changes were evident in that patient. In the remaining three patients, no symptom progression or change was apparent. None of the patients exhibited new symptoms, or any increase in the symptoms of constipation, obstipation, or impaction.

7. Summary, discussion, and conclusions

One of the consequences of greater worldwide longevity has been an upsurge in the number of older adults living with neurocognitive disease [1, 2]. Currently, over 50 million people in the world have neurocognitive diseases, almost 20 million of which have Parkinson's Disease (PD) or Neurocognitive Disorder with Lewy Bodies (NCDLB). The overall number of people in the world with neurocognitive disease is expected to exceed 131.5 million by year 2050, with about 43 million of those attributable to PC or NCDLB [1, 2, 4, 5].

In 2015, the global cost of providing treatment and long-term care to people with neurocognitive disease was about $818 billion. That figure is expected to exceed $4 trillion by year 2050 [2–4]. The cost of providing treatment and long-term care to patients with PD and NCDLB exceeds one third of the total global expense, because Lewy body diseases like PD and NCDLB encompass a large and varied number of cognitive, motor, and autonomic symptoms [8]. Lewy bodies are abnormal intracellular aggregations of α-synuclein protein [9] that can affect any neurotransmitter pathway in any one or all of the ANS, CNS, PNS, or ENS.

Gastric slowing due to α-synucleopathology is an almost universal feature of PD and NCDLB, but is often not a focus of treatment [18]. As the symptoms of constipation, obstipation, and impaction progress, they negatively impact mobility, sleep, cognition, and mood, increasing the cost of care and debilitating or dramatically reducing the quality of life for patients [11–17]. From a phylogenetic perspective, the central nervous system and all its higher cortical functions exist solely in service of the alimentary canal. The impact that constipation, obstipation, and impaction have on the quality of life cannot be overstated.

When constipation, obstipation, and impaction are addressed for patients with α-synucleopathology, conventional over-the-counter treatments are usually recommended, even though research has shown that such treatments are ineffective for patients with PD and NCDLB [12]. Such treatment suggests unawareness that constipation is considered a common feature of α-synucleopathology, likely prodromal for Lewy body (α-synuclein) pathology, often manifesting years before other α-synucleopathology [17, 21, 37, 54–57]; and that in constellation with late-life onset depression, cognitive impairment, and RBD/RSWA, constipation may be a reliable biomarker for α-synucleopathology [18, 24, 25, 29, 30].

In this chapter, a description was given of α-synucleopathology in the Lewy body diseases PD and NCDLB, and its symptomatic manifestations in the ENS. Explanation was made for the specific mechanisms through which α-synucleopathology interferes with gastric motility, as well as the specific mechanisms through which specific medications can address α-synucleopathology in the ENS. It was hypothesized that α-synuclein pathological impairment of the MP and CSMP in patients with NCDLB and PD might be mitigated with the use of the AchEI donepezil, which has demonstrated effectiveness for boosting cholinergic activity, and mitigating symptoms of α-synucleopathology in patients with PD and NCDLB. The expected outcomes included reduction of the symptoms of constipation, obstipation, and impaction. It was also hypothesized that donepezil might have specific benefit for reducing constipation in PD and NCDLB patients for whom L-dopa agents like carbidopa-levodopa are prescribed.

A series of case studies was then presented, in which four patients at varying levels of disease progression with PD and NCDLB were orally administered donepezil in daily doses varying from 5 to 10 mg. Results indicated that the use of donepezil was associated with significant reduction in the symptoms of constipation, obstipation and/or impaction. Although there had been progression of cognitive interference, movement disorders, and other Lewy body pathology in two of the patients (case studies #3 and #4), symptom reduction for constipation, obstipation and/or impaction for all four patients was consistent over time, assessed at intervals of two, four and 6 weeks, and later, at intervals of 6, 12, and 18 months [135–137].

The findings support the hypothesis donepezil might reduce α-synuclein pathological impairment of the MP and CSMP in patients with NCDLB and PD, increasing bowel motility and reducing the symptom of constipation. The findings also support the hypothesis that donepezil might have specific benefit in reducing constipation in PD and NCDLB patients for whom L-dopa agents like carbidopa-levodopa are prescribed. It appears that donepezil achieves such symptom reduction through its "dual action:" in part, specifically and reversibly limiting the action of the acetylcholine-hydrolyzing enzyme acetylcholinesterase [129, 130]; and in part, by independently facilitating neuronal nicotinic acetylcholine receptors [131]. The combined effect of these two mechanisms is to effectively increase acetylcholine levels and mitigate the symptoms of cholinergic impairment [128].

The reduction of constipation, obstipation, and impaction without exacerbation or emergence of other symptoms in all four patients over an 18 month period suggests that donepezil might be efficacious for treating these symptoms over an extended time frame, including its use for patients simultaneously taking carbidopa-levodopa. The findings are also consistent with previous research demonstrating that donepezil is effective for slowing or reversing cognitive symptom progression in Lewy body disorders, including short-term memory loss, difficulty with word-finding, hallucinations, and cognitive interference [107, 110–123]. To increase our understanding of α-synucleopathology and its role in PD and NCDLB, the symptoms of constipation, obstipation, and impaction, and effective medical interventions, further research is suggested, including longitudinal case studies, as well as large data set analyses using larger numbers of subjects matched for diagnosis, age, gender, and other variables.

8. Declarations

This research received no specific grant from any funding agency in the public, commercial, or not-for-profit sectors. Written consent was provided by each of the four patients described in the case studies to release the clinical information contained therein. Patient identifiers have been kept to a minimum. This paper was written according to the Ethical Principles of the American Psychological Association. Charles M. Lepkowsky, PhD, is the sole author of this work, including its conception and design; the acquisition, analysis, and interpretation of data; drafting, writing, and editing; and final approval of the version published; and accepts accountability for all aspects of the work in ensuring that questions related to the accuracy or integrity of any part of the work are appropriately investigated and resolved.

Conflict of interest

There are no competing interests involved in the research reported or the writing of this chapter.

Author details

Charles M. Lepkowsky
Independent Practice, Solvang, CA, USA

*Address all correspondence to: clepkowsky@gmail.com

References

[1] World Health Organization. Life expectancy: Global Health Observatory Data [Internet]. 2018. Available from: http://www.who.int/gho/mortality_burden_disease/life_tables/situation_trends/en/ [Accessed 2018-07-08]

[2] US Census Bureau. An Aging World: 2015 [Internet]. 2016. Available from: https://www.census.gov/content/dam/Census/library/publications/2016/demo/p95-16-1.pdf [Accessed 2018-07-08]

[3] Alzheimer's Disease International. World Alzheimer Report 2015: The Global Impact of Dementia: An Analysis of Prevalence, Incidence, Cost and Trends [Internet]. 2016. Available from: https://www.alz.co.uk/research/WorldAlzheimerReport2015.pdf [Accessed 2018-07-08]

[4] Kowal S, Dall T, Chakrabarti R, Storm M, Jain A. The current and projected economic burden of Parkinson's disease in the United States. Movement Disorders. 2013;**28**(3):311-318. DOI: 10.1002/mds.25292

[5] Hebert LE, Weuve J, Scherr PA, Evans DA. Alzheimer disease in the United States (2010-2050) estimated using the 2010 census. Neurology. 2013;**80**(19):1778-1783. DOI: 10.1212/WNL.0b013e31828726f5

[6] U.S. Centers for Medicare and Medicaid Services. Hospice Center [Internet]. 2015. Available from: http://www.cms.gov/Medicare/MedicareFee-for-Service-Payment/Hospice/Medicare_Hospice_Data.html.[Accessed 2016-07-12]

[7] U.S. Burden of Disease Collaborators. The state of U.S. health, 1990-2010: Burden of diseases, injuries, and risk factors. JAMA. 2013;**310**(6):591-608. DOI: 10.1001/jama.2013.13805

[8] Lepkowsky CM. Neurocognitive disorder with Lewy bodies: Evidence-based diagnosis and treatment. Practice Innovations. 2016;**1**(4):234-242. DOI: 10.1037/pri0000031

[9] Taguchi K, Watanabe Y, Tsujimura A, Tanaka M. Brain region-dependent differential expression of alpha-synuclein. The Journal of Comparative Neurology. 2015;**524**(6):1236-1258. DOI: 10.1002/cne.23901. [Accessed 2018-07-08]

[10] Sanjari MH, Zare-Shahabadi A, Rahmani F, Rezaei N. Neurotransmission systems in Parkinson's disease. Reviews in the Neurosciences. 2017;**28**(5):509-536. DOI: 10.1515/revneuro-2016-0068

[11] Gonera E, Van't Hof M, Berger H, van Weel C, Horstink M. Symptoms and duration of the prodromal phase in Parkinson's disease. Movement Disorders. 1997;**12**(6):871-876. DOI: 10.1002/mds.870120607

[12] Phillips C, Polakoff D, Maue S, Mauch R. Assessment of constipation management in long-term care patients. Journal of the American Medical Directors Association. 2001;**2**(4):149-154. PMID: 12812571

[13] Klockgether T. Parkinson's disease: Clinical aspects. Cell and Tissue Research. 2004;**318**(1):115-120. DOI: 10.1007/s00441-004-0975-6

[14] Chaudhuri K, Healy D, Schapira A. Non-motor symptoms of Parkinson's disease: Diagnosis and management. Lancet Neurology. 2006;**5**(3):235-245. DOI: 10.1016/S1474-4422(06)70373-8

[15] Winter Y, von Campenhausen S, Brozova H, Skoupa J, Reese J, Bötzel K, et al. Costs of Parkinson's disease in Eastern Europe: A Czech cohort study. Parkinsonism & Related Disorders.

2010;**16**(1):51-56. DOI: 10.1016/j.parkreldis.2009.07.005

[16] Wasner G, Deuschl G. Pains in Parkinson disease—Many syndromes under one umbrella. Nature Reviews. Neurology. 2012;**8**(5):284-294. DOI: 10.1038/nrneurol.2012.54

[17] Rossi M, Merello M, Perez-Lloret S. Management of constipation in Parkinson's disease. Expert Opinion on Pharmacotherapy. 2014;**16**(4):547-557. DOI: 10.1517/14656566.2015.997211

[18] Lepkowsky CM. Donepezil for Lewy body constipation: Four case studies. Activitas Nervosa Superior. 2017;**59**(1):19-27. DOI: 10.1007/s41470-017-0004-1

[19] Scott D, Roy S. α-Synuclein inhibits intersynaptic vesicle mobility and maintains recycling-pool homeostasis. The Journal of Neuroscience. 2012;**32**(30):10129-10135. DOI: 10.1523/JNEUROSCI.0535-12.2012

[20] Larson M, Sherman M, Greimel S, Kuskowski M, Schneider J, Bennett D, et al. Soluble α-synuclein is a novel modulator of Alzheimer's disease pathophysiology. The Journal of Neuroscience. 2012;**32**(30):10253-10266. DOI: 10.1523/JNEUROSCI.0581-12.2012

[21] Donaghy P, McKeith I. The clinical characteristics of dementia with Lewy bodies and a consideration of prodromal diagnosis. Alzheimer's Research & Therapy. 2014;**6**(4):46. DOI: 10.1186/alzrt274. [Internet]. Available from: https://alzres.biomedcentral.com/articles/10.1186/alzrt274 [Accessed 2016-06-13]

[22] McKeith I, Dickson D, Lowe J, Emre M, O'Brien J, Feldman H, et al. Consortium on DLB. Diagnosis and management of dementia with Lewy bodies: Third report of the DLB consortium. Neurology. 2005;**65**(12):1863-1872. DOI: 10.1212/01.wnl.0000187889.17253.b1

[23] McKeith IG. Consensus guidelines for the clinical and pathologic diagnosis of dementia with Lewy bodies (DLB): Report of the consortium on DLB international workshop. Journal of Alzheimer's Disease. 2006;**9**(3 Suppl):417-423. PMID: 16914880

[24] McCarter SJ, St Louis EK, Boeve BF. REM sleep behavior disorder and REM sleep without Atonia as an early manifestation of degenerative neurological disease. Current Neurology and Neuroscience Reports. 2012;**12**(2):182-192. DOI: 10.1007/s11910-012-0253-z

[25] Allan LM, Ballard CG, Allen J, Murray A, Davidson AW, McKeith I, et al. Autonomic dysfunction in dementia. Journal of Neurology, Neurosurgery, and Psychiatry. 2007;**78**(7):671-677. DOI: 10.1136/jnnp.2006.102343

[26] Cersosimo M. Gastrointestinal biopsies for the diagnosis of alpha-synuclein pathology in Parkinson's disease. Gastroenterology Research and Practice. 2015: Article ID 476041. DOI: 10.1155/2015/476041 [. Accessed 2016-06-17]

[27] Funabe S, Takao M, Saito Y, Hatsuta H, Sugiyama M, Ito S, et al. Neuropathologic analysis of Lewy-related α-synucleinopathy in olfactory mucosa. Neuropathology. 2013;**33**(1):47-58. DOI: 10.1111/j.1440-1789.2012.01329.x

[28] Landy KM, Salmon DP, Galasko D, Filoteo JV, Festa EK, Heindel WC, et al. Motion discrimination in dementia with Lewy bodies and Alzheimer disease. Neurology. 2015;**85**(16):1376-1382. DOI: 10.1212/WNL.0000000000002028

[29] Kosaka K, Oyanagi S, Matsushita M, Hori A. Presenile dementia with Alzheimer-, Pick- and Lewy-body changes. Acta Neuropathologica. 1976;**36**(3):221-233. . PMID: 188300. DOI: 10.1007/BF00685366

[30] Ferman TJ, Smith GE, Kantarci K, Boeve BF, Pankratz VS, Dickson DW, et al. Nonamnestic mild cognitive impairment progresses to dementia with Lewy bodies. Neurology. 2013;**81**(23):2032-2038. DOI: 10.1212/01.wnl.0000436942.55281.47

[31] Molloy S, McKeith IG, O'Brien JT, Burn DJ. The role of levodopa in the management of dementia with Lewy bodies. Journal of Neurology, Neurosurgery, and Psychiatry. 2005;**76**(9):1200-1203. DOI: 10.1136/jnnp.2004.052332

[32] Schenck C, Boeve BF, Mahowald MW. Delayed emergence of a parkinsonian disorder or dementia in 81% of older men initially diagnosed with idiopathic rapid eye movement sleep behavior disorder: A 16-year update on a previously reported series. Sleep Medicine;**14**(8):744-748. DOI: 10.1016/j.sleep.2012.10.009

[33] Coune PG, Craveiro M, Gaugler MN, Mlynárik V, Schneider BL, Aebischer P, et al. An in vivo ultrahigh field 14.1 T (1) H-MRS study on 6-OHDA and α-synuclein-based rat models of Parkinson's disease: GABA as an early disease marker. NMR in Biomedicine. 2013;**26**(1):43-50. DOI: 10.1002/nbm.2817.

[34] Kupsky WJ, Grimes MM, Sweeting J, Bertsch R, Cote LJ. Parkinson's disease and megacolon: Concentric hyaline inclusions (Lewy bodies) in enteric ganglion cells. Neurology. 1987;**37**(7):1253-1255. PMID: 3037441

[35] Shankle WR, Landing BH, Ang SM, Chui H, Villarreal-Engelhardt G, Zarow C. Studies of the enteric nervous system in Alzheimer disease and other dementias of the elderly: Enteric neurons in Alzheimer disease. Modern Pathology. 1993;**6**(1):10-14. PMID: 8426853

[36] Braak H, Braak E. Pathoanatomy of Parkinson's disease. Journal of Neurology. 2000;**247**(Supplement 2):ii3-ii10. DOI: 10.1007/PL00007758

[37] Abbott R, Webster R, Petrovitch H, Tanner C, Davis D, Masaki K, et al. Bowel movement frequency in late-life and incidental Lewy bodies. Movement Disorders. 2007;**2**(11):1581-1586. DOI: 10.1002/mds.21560

[38] Lebouvier T, Chaumette T, Paillusson S, Duyckaerts C, Bruley des Varannes S, Neunlist M, et al. The second brain and Parkinson's disease. The European Journal of Neuroscience. 2009;**30**(5):735-741. DOI: 10.1111/j.1460-9568.2009.06873.x

[39] Beach T, Adler C, Sue L, Vedders L, Lue L, White C, et al. Multi-organ distribution of phosphorylated α-synuclein histopathology in subjects with Lewy body disorders. Acta Neuropathologica. 2010;**119**(6):689-702. DOI: 10.1007/s00401-010-0664-3

[40] Lebouvier T, Neunlist M, Bruley d, Varannes S, Coron E, Drouard A, et al. Colonic biopsies to assess the neuropathology of Parkinson's disease and its relationship with symptoms. PLoS One. 2010;**5**(9):e12728. DOI: 10.1371/journal.pone.0012728

[41] Gold A, Turkalp Z, Munoz D. Enteric alpha-synuclein expression is increased in Parkinson's disease but not Alzheimer's disease. Movement Disorders. 2013;**28**(2):237-241. DOI: 10.1002/mds.25298

[42] Semar S, Klotz M, Letiembre M, Van Ginneken C, Braun A, Jost V, et al. Changes of the enteric nervous system in amyloid-β protein precursor transgenic mice correlate with disease progression. Journal of Alzheimer's Disease. 2013;**36**(1):7-20. DOI: 10.3233/JAD-120511

[43] Gelpi E, Navarro-Otano J, Tolosa E, Gaig C, Compta Y, Rey M, et al. Multiple organ involvement by alpha-synuclein

pathology in Lewy body disorders. Movement Disorders. 2014;**29**(8):1010-1018. DOI: 10.1002/mds.25776

[44] Corbillé A, Neunlist M, Derkinderen P. Cross-linking for the analysis of α-synuclein in the enteric nervous system. Journal of Neurochemistry. 2016;**139**(5):839-847. DOI: 10.1111/jnc.13845

[45] Jost W, Schimrigk K. Constipation in Parkinson's disease. Klinische Wochenschrift. 1991;**69**(20):906-909. Available from: https://link.springer.com/article/10.1007/BF01798536 [Accessed 2016-01-04]

[46] Tanaka Y, Kato T, Nishida H, Yamada M, Koumura A, Sakurai T, et al. Is there a delayed gastric emptying of patients with early-stage, untreated Parkinson's disease? An analysis using the 13C-acetate breath test. Journal of Neurology. 2011;**258**(3):421-426. DOI: 10.1007/s00415-010-5769-z

[47] Kaye J, Gage H, Kimber A, Storey L, Trend P. Excess burden of constipation in Parkinson's disease: A pilot study. Movement Disorders. 2006;**21**(8):1270-1273. DOI: 10.1002/mds.20942

[48] Martinez-Martin P, Schapira AH, Stocchi F, Sethi K, Odin P, MacPhee G, et al. Prevalence of nonmotor symptoms in Parkinson's disease in an international setting; study using nonmotor symptoms questionnaire in 545 patients. Movement Disorders. 2007;**22**(11):1623-1629. DOI: 10.1002/mds.21586

[49] Langston J. The Parkinson's complex: Parkinsonism is just the tip of the iceberg. Annals of Neurology. 2006;**59**(4):591-596. DOI: 10.1002/ana.20834

[50] Dickson DW, Fujishiro H, Delle Donne A, Menke J, Ahmed Z, Klos KJ, et al. Evidence that incidental Lewy body disease is pre-symptomatic Parkinson's disease. Acta Neuropathologica. 2008;**115**(4):437-444. DOI: 10.1007/s00401-008-0345-7.

[51] Fasano A, Visanji NP, Liu LW, Lang AE, Pfeiffer RF. Gastrointestinal dysfunction in Parkinson's disease. Lancet Neurology. 2015;**14**(6):625-639. DOI: 10.1016/S1474-4422(15)00007-1.

[52] Visanji N, Marras C. The relevance of pre-motor symptoms in Parkinson's disease. Expert Review of Neurotherapeutics. 2015;**15**(10):1205-1217. DOI: 10.1586/14737175.2015.1083423

[53] Schulz J, Hausmann L, Hardy J. 199 years of Parkinson disease – What have we learned and what is the path to the future? Journal of Neurochemistry. 2016;**139**(S1):3-7. DOI: 10.1111/jnc.13733

[54] Pfeiffer R. Gastrointestinal dysfunction in Parkinson's disease. Lancet Neurology. 2003;**2**(2):107-116. PMID: 12849267

[55] Savica R, Carlin J, Grossardt B, Bower J, Ahlskog J, Maraganore D, et al. Medical records documentation of constipation preceding Parkinson disease: A case-control study. Neurology. 2009;**73**(21):1752-1758. DOI: 10.1212/WNL.0b013e3181c34af5

[56] Iranzo A, Gelpi E, Tolosa E, Molinuevo J, Serradell M, Gaig C, et al. Neuropathology of prodromal Lewy body disease. Movement Disorders. 2014;**29**(3):410-415. DOI: 10.1002/mds.25825

[57] Alzforum. International Dementia with Lewy Bodies Conference 2015 [Internet]. Available from: http://www.alzforum.org/print-series/554861. [Accessed 2016-01-03]

[58] Wakabayashi K, Takahashi H, Takeda S, Ohama E, Ikuta F. Lewy bodies in the enteric nervous system in Parkinson's disease. Archives of Histology and Cytology.

1989;**52**(Supplement P):191-194. [Internet] Available from: https://pdfs.semanticscholar.org/d2c8/68f7e2853ec299d7962dd75048ac239d3d48.pdf [Accessed 2016-03-15]

[59] Braaka H, de Vosb R, Bohlc J, Del Tredici K. Gastric α-synuclein immunoreactive inclusions in Meissner's and Auerbach's plexuses in cases staged for Parkinson's disease-related brain pathology. Neuroscience Letters. 2006;**396**(1):67-72. DOI: 10.1016/j.neulet.2005.11.012

[60] Hawkes C, Del Tredici K, Braak H. Parkinson's disease: A dual-hit hypothesis. Neuropathology and Applied Neurobiology. 2007;**33**(6):599-614. DOI: 10.1111/j.1365-2990.2007.00874.x

[61] Minguez-Castellanos A, Chamorro C, Escamilla-Sevilla F, Ortega-Moreno A, Rebollo A, Gomez-Rio M, et al. Do α-synuclein aggregates in autonomic plexuses predate Lewy body disorders? Neurology. 2007;**68**(23):2012-2018. DOI: 10.1212/01.wnl.0000264429.59379.d9

[62] Holmqvist S, Chutna O, Bousset L, Aldrin-Kirk P, Li W, Björklund T, et al. Direct evidence of Parkinson pathology spread from the gastrointestinal tract to the brain in rats. Acta Neurologica Scandinavica. 2014;**128**(6):805-820. DOI: 10.1007/s00401-014-1343-6

[63] Gjerløff T, Fedorova T, Knudsen K, Munk O, Nahimi A, Jacobsen S, et al. Imaging acetylcholinesterase density in peripheral organs in Parkinson's disease with 11C-donepezil PET. Brain. 2015;**138**(3):653-663. DOI: 10.1093/brain/awu369

[64] Porter A, Wattchow D, Brookes S, Costa M. Cholinergic and nitrergic interneurones in the myenteric plexus of the human colon. Gut. 2002;**51**(1):70-75. DOI: 10.1136/gut.51.1.70

[65] McKeith I, Galasko D, Kosaka K, Perry E, Dickson D, Hansen L, et al. Consensus guidelines for the clinical and pathologic diagnosis of dementia with Lewy bodies (DLB): Report of the consortium on DLB international workshop. Neurology. 1996;**47**(5):1113-1124. DOI: 10.1212/WNL.47.5.1113

[66] Smith WW, Jiang H, Pei Z, Tanaka Y, Morita H, Sawa A, et al. Endoplasmic reticulum stress and mitochondrial cell death pathways mediate A53T mutant alpha-synuclein-induced toxicity. Human Molecular Genetics. 2005;**14**(24):3801-3811. DOI: 10.1093/hmg/ddi396

[67] Cooper AA, Gitler AD, Cashikar A, Haynes CM, Hill KJ, Bhullar B, et al. Alpha-synuclein blocks ER-Golgi traffic and Rab1 rescues neuron loss in Parkinson's models. Science. 2006;**313**(5785):324-328. DOI: 10.1126/science.1129462

[68] Devi L, Anandatheerthavarada HK. Mitochondrial trafficking of APP and alpha synuclein: Relevance to mitochondrial dysfunction in Alzheimer's and Parkinson's diseases. Biochimica et Biophysica Acta (BBA) - Molecular Basis of Disease. 2010;**1802**(1):11-19. DOI: 10.1016/j.bbadis.2009.07.007

[69] Parsons CG, Danysz W, Dekundy A, Pulte I. Memantine and cholinesterase inhibitors: Complementary mechanisms in the treatment of Alzheimer's disease. Neurotoxicity Research. 2013;**24**(3):358-369. DOI: 10.1007/s12640-013-9398-z], 10.1007/s12640-013-9398-z]

[70] Edwards L, Quigley E, Pfeiffer R. Gastrointestinal dysfunction in Parkinson's disease: Frequency and pathophysiology. Neurology. 1992;**42**(4):726-732. DOI: 10.1212/WNL.42.4.726

[71] Johanson J, Sonnenberg A, Koch T, McCarty D. Association of constipation with neurologic diseases. Digestive Diseases and Sciences. 1992;**37**(2):179-186. PMID: 1735333

[72] Winge K, Rasmussen D, Werdelin L. Constipation in neurological diseases. Journal of Neurology, Neurosurgery, and Psychiatry. 2003;**74**(1):13-19. DOI: 10.1136/jnnp.74.1.13

[73] Sveinbjornsdottir S. The clinical symptoms of Parkinson's disease. Journal of Neurochemistry. 2016;**139**(S1):318-324. DOI: 10.1111/jnc.13691

[74] Lebouvier T, Tasselli M, Paillusson S, Pouclet H, Neunlist M, Derkinderen P. Biopsable neural tissues: Toward new biomarkers for Parkinson's disease? Frontiers in Psychiatry. 2010;**1**:128. DOI: 10.3389/fpsyt.2010.00128. [Internet] Available from: https://www.frontiersin.org/articles/10.3389/fpsyt.2010.00128/full [Accessed 2016-01-14]

[75] Molloy S, McKeith I, O'Brien J, Burn D. The role of levodopa in the management of dementia with Lewy bodies. Journal of Neurology, Neurosurgery, and Psychiatry. 2005;**76**(9):200-1203. DOI: 10.1136/jnnp.2004.052332

[76] Lepkowsky CM. Medications linked to cognitive impairment in older adults. Practice Innovations. 2016;**1**(4):253-264. DOI: 10.1037/pri0000033

[77] Merck Pharmaceuticals: Product Information: Sinemet CR (carbidopa-levodopa). [Internet]. 2016. Available from: https://www.merck.com/product/usa/pi_circulars/s/sinemet/sinemet_pi.pdf [Accessed 2016-01-15]

[78] Boustani M, Campbell N, Munger S, Maidment I, Fox C. Impact of anticholinergics on the aging brain: A review and practical application. Aging Health. 2008;**4**(3):311-320. DOI: 10.2217/1745509X.4.3.311

[79] Campbell N, Boustani M, Limbil T, Ott C, Fox C, Maidment I, et al. The cognitive impact of anticholinergics: A clinical review. Clinical Interventions in Aging. 2009;**4**(1):225-233. PMID: 19554093 PMCID: PMC2697587

[80] Cai X, Campbell N, Khan B, Callahan C, Boustani M. Long-term anticholinergic use and the aging brain. Alzheimer's & Dementia: The Journal of the Alzheimer's Association. 2013;**9**(4):377-385. DOI: 10.1016/j.jalz.2012.02.005

[81] Hutchinson M, Fazzini E. Cholinesterase inhibition in Parkinson's disease. Journal of Neurology, Neurosurgery, and Psychiatry. 1996;**61**(3):324-325. PMID: 8795611 PMCID: PMC486563

[82] Tiraboschi P, Hansen L, Alford M, Sabbagh M, Schoos B, Masliah E, et al. Cholinergic dysfunction in diseases with Lewy bodies. Neurology. 2000;**54**(2):407-411. PMID: 10668703

[83] Francis P, Perry E. Cholinergic and other neurotransmitter mechanisms in Parkinson's disease, Parkinson's disease dementia, and dementia with Lewy bodies. Movement Disorders. 2007;**22**(S17):S351-S357. DOI: 10.1002/mds.21683

[84] Bohnen N, Albin R. The cholinergic system and Parkinson disease. Behavioural Brain Research. 2011;**221**(2):564-573. DOI: 10.1016/j.bbr.2009.12.048

[85] Müller M, Bohnen N. Cholinergic dysfunction in Parkinson's disease. Current Neurology and Neuroscience Reports. 2013;**13**(9):377. DOI: 10.1007/s11910-013-0377-9

[86] Grothe M, Schuster C, Bauer F, Heinsen H, Prudlo J, Teipel S. Atrophy of the cholinergic basal forebrain in dementia with Lewy bodies and Alzheimer's disease dementia. Journal of Neurology. 2014;**261**(10):1939-1948. DOI: 10.1007/s00415-014-7439-z

[87] Hall H, Reyes S, Landeck N, Bye C, Leanza G, Double K, et al. Hippocampal Lewy pathology and cholinergic dysfunction are associated with dementia in Parkinson's disease. Brain. 2014;**137**(9):2493-2508. DOI: 10.1093/brain/awu193

[88] Perez-Lloret S, Barrantes F. Deficits in cholinergic neurotransmission and their clinical correlates in Parkinson's disease. Npj Parkinson's Disease. 2016;**2**,. Article number: 16001. DOI: 10.1038/npjparkd.2016.1

[89] Scharre D, Chang S, Nagaraja H, Park A, Adeli A, Agrawal P, et al. Paired studies comparing clinical profiles of Lewy body dementia with Alzheimer's and Parkinson's diseases. Journal of Alzheimer's Disease. 2016;**549**(3):995-1004. DOI: 10.3233/JAD-160384

[90] Watanabe H, Ieda T, Katayama T, Takeda A, Aiba I, Doyu M, et al. Cardiac (123)Imetaiodobenzylguanidine (MIBG) uptake in dementia with Lewy bodies: Comparison with Alzheimer's disease. Journal of Neurology, Neurosurgery, and Psychiatry. 2001;**70**(6):781-783. [Internet] available from: http://jnnp.bmj.com/ [Accessed on 2017-12-15]

[91] Perry E, Smith C, Court J, Perry R. Cholinergic nicotinic and muscarinic receptors in dementia of Alzheimer, Parkinson and Lewy body types. Journal of Neurology. 1990;**2**(3):149-158. PMID: 2175197

[92] McKeith IG. Spectrum of Parkinson's disease, Parkinson's dementia, and Lewy body dementia. Neurologic Clinics. 2000;**18**:865-902. PMID: 11072265

[93] Aarsland D, Hutchinson M, Larsen J. Cognitive, psychiatric and motor response to galantamine in Parkinson's disease with dementia. International Journal of Geriatric Psychiatry. 2003;**18**(10):937-941. DOI: 10.1002/gps.949

[94] Folstein MF, Folstein SE, McHugh P. Mini-mental state: A practical method for grading the cognitive state of patients for the clinician. Journal of Psychiatric Research. 1975;**12**(3):189-198. PMID: 1202204

[95] McKeith I, Del Ser T, Spano P, Emre M, Wesnes K, Anand R, et al. Efficacy of rivastigmine in dementia with Lewy bodies: A randomised, double-blind, placebo-controlled international study. Lancet. 2000;**356**(9247):2031-2036. DOI: 10.1016/S0140-6736(00)03399-7

[96] McKeith IG, Grace JB, Walker Z, Byrne EJ, Wilkinson D, Stevens T, et al. Rivastigmine in the treatment of dementia with Lewy bodies: Preliminary findings from an open trial. International Journal of Geriatric Psychiatry. 2000;**15**(5):387-392. PMID: 10822236

[97] Grace J, Daniel S, Stevens T, Shankar KK, Walker Z, Byrne EJ, et al. Long-term use of rivastigmine in patients with dementia with Lewy bodies: An open-label trial. International Psychogeriatrics. 2001;**13**(2):199-205. PMID: 11495394

[98] Bullock R, Cameron A. Rivastigmine for the treatment of dementia and visual hallucinations associated with Parkinson's disease: A case series. Current Medical Research and Opinion. 2002;**18**(5):258-264. DOI: 10.1185/030079902125000813

[99] Emre M, Aarsland D, Albanese A, Byrne EJ, Deuschl G, De Deyn PP, et al. Rivastigmine for dementia associated with Parkinson's disease. The New England Journal of Medicine. 2004;**351**(24):2509-2518. DOI: 10.1056/NEJMoa041470

[100] Bourke D, Druckenbrod RW. Possible association between donepezil and worsening Parkinson's disease. The Annals of Pharmacotherapy. 1998;**32**(5):610-611. DOI: 10.1345/aph.17355

[101] Babic T, Zurak N. Convulsions induced by donepezil. Journal of Neurology, Neurosurgery, and Psychiatry. 1999;**66**(3):410. PMID 1008455

[102] Hashimoto M, Imamura T, Tanimukai S, Kazui H, Mori E. Urinary incontinence: An unrecognized adverse effect with donepezil. Lancet. 2000;**356**(9229):568. DOI: 10.1016/S0140-6736(00)02588-5

[103] Onofrj M, Thomas A. Severe worsening of parkinsonism in Lewy body dementia due to donepezil. Neurology. 2003;**61**(10):1452. DOI: 10.1212/01.WNL.0000094201.80888.DA

[104] Rozzini L, Ghianda D, Trabucchi M, Padovani A. Severe worsening of parkinsonism in Lewy body dementia due to donepezil. Neurology. 2004;**63**(8):1543-1544. PMID: 15505196

[105] Iraqi A, Hughes T. An unusual case of nightmares with galantamine. Journal of the American Geriatrics Society. 2009;**57**(3):565. DOI: 10.1111/j.1532-5415.2009.02157.x

[106] News Medical: Health News and Information: Alzheimer's Drug Aricept (donepezil) Linked to Serious Side Effects. [1]. 2015. Available from: http://www.news-medical.net/news/20150121/Alzheimers-drug-Aricept-(donepezil)-linked-to-serious-side-effects.aspx. [Accessed: 2016-01-15]

[107] Fabbrini G, Barbanti P, Aurilia C, Pauletti C, Lenzi GL, Meco G. Donepezil in the treatment of hallucinations and delusions in Parkinson's disease. Neurological Sciences. 2002;**23**(1):41-43. DOI: 10.1007/s100720200022

[108] Bergman J, Lerner V. Successful use of donepezil for the treatment of psychotic symptoms in patients with Parkinson's disease. Clinical Neuropharmacology. 2002;**25**(2):107-110. PMID: 11981238

[109] Shea C, MacKnight C, Rockwood K. Donepezil for treatment of dementia with Lewy bodies: A case series of nine patients. International Psychogeriatrics. 1998;**10**(3):229-238. PMID: 9785144

[110] Aarsland D, Brønnick K, Karlsen K. Donepezil for dementia with Lewy bodies: A case study. International Journal of Geriatric Psychiatry. 1999;**14**(1):69-72. PMID: 10029938

[111] Samuel W, Caligiuri M, Galasko D, Lacro J, Marini M, McClure FS, et al. Better cognitive and psychopathologic response to donepezil in patients prospectively diagnosed as dementia with Lewy bodies: A preliminary study. International Journal of Geriatric Psychiatry. 2000;**15**(9):794-802. PMID: 10984725

[112] Rojas-Fernandez CH. Successful use of donepezil for the treatment of dementia with Lewy bodies. The Annals of Pharmacotherapy. 2001;**35**(2):202-205. DOI: 10.1345/aph.10192

[113] Aarsland D, Laake K, Larsen J, Janvin C. Donepezil for cognitive impairment in Parkinson's disease: A randomised controlled study. Journal of Neurology, Neurosurgery, and Psychiatry. 2002;**72**:708-712. DOI: 10.1136/jnnp.72.6.708

[114] Aarsland D, Mosimann UP, McKeith IG. Role of cholinesterase inhibitors in Parkinson's disease and dementia with Lewy bodies. Journal of Geriatric Psychiatry and Neurology. 2004;**17**(3):164-171. DOI: 10.1177/0891988704267463

[115] Leroi I, Brandt J, Reich SG, Lyketsos CG, Grill S, Thompson R, et al. Randomized placebo-controlled trial of donepezil in cognitive impairment in Parkinson's disease. International Journal of Geriatric Psychiatry. 2004;**19**(1):1-8. DOI: 10.1002/gps.993

[116] McKeith I, Mintzer J, Aarsland D, Burn D, Chiu H, Cohen-Mansfield J, et al. International psychogeriatric association expert meeting on DLB. Dementia with Lewy bodies. Lancet Neurology. 2004;**3**(1):19-28. PMID: 14693108

[117] Thomas AJ, Burn DJ, Rowan EN, Littlewood E, Newby J, Cousins D, et al. A comparison of the efficacy of donepezil in Parkinson's disease with dementia and dementia with Lewy bodies. International Journal of Geriatric Psychiatry. 2005;**20**(10):938-944. DOI: 10.1002/gps.1381

[118] Ravina B, Putt M, Siderow A, Farrar J, Gillespie M, Crawley A, et al. Donepezil for dementia in Parkinson's disease: A randomised, double blind, placebo controlled, crossover study. Journal of Neurology, Neurosurgery, and Psychiatry. 2005;**76**(7):934-939. DOI: 10.1136/jnnp.2004.050682

[119] Ikeda M, Mori E, Kosaka K, Iseki E, Hashimoto M, Matsukawa N, et al. Donepezil-DLB study investigators. Long-term safety and efficacy of donepezil in patients with dementia with Lewy bodies: Results from a 52-week, open-label, multicenter extension study. Dementia and Geriatric Cognitive Disorders. 2013;**36**(3-4):229-241. DOI: 10.1159/000351672

[120] Ikeda M, Mori E, Matsuo K, Nakagawa M, Kosaka K. Donepezil for dementia with Lewy bodies: A randomized, placebo-controlled, confirmatory phase III trial. Alzheimer's Research & Therapy. 2015;7(1):4. DOI: 10.1186/s13195-014-0083-0

[121] Rolinski M, Fox C, Maidment I, McShane R. Cholinesterase inhibitors for dementia with Lewy bodies, Parkinson's disease dementia and cognitive impairment in Parkinson's disease. Cochrane Database of Systematic Reviews. 2012;(3):CD006504. DOI: 10.1002/14651858.CD006504.pub2

[122] Bosboom JL, Stoffers D, Wolters ECH. Cognitive dysfunction and dementia in Parkinson's disease. Journal of Neural Transmission (Vienna). 2004;**111**(10-11):1303-1315. DOI: 10.1007/s00702-004-0168-1

[123] Birks J. Cholinesterase inhibitors for Alzheimer's disease. Cochrane Database of Systematic Reviews. 2006;**1**:CD005593. DOI: 10.1002/14651858.CD005593

[124] Minett TSC, Thomas A, Wilkinson L, Daniel SL, Sanders J, Richardson J, et al. What happens when donepezil is suddenly withdrawn? An open label trial in dementia with Lewy bodies and Parkinson's disease with dementia. International Journal of Geriatric Psychiatry. 2003;**18**(11):988-993. DOI: 10.1002/gps.995

[125] Mori E, Iked M, Kosaka K. Donepezil for dementia with Lewy bodies: A randomized, placebo controlled trial. Annals of Neurology. 2012;**72**(1):41-52. DOI: 10.1002/ana.23557

[126] Mori E, Ikeda M, Nagai R, Matsuo K, Nakagawa M, Kosaka K. Long-term donepezil use for dementia with Lewy bodies: Results from an open-label extension of phase III trial. Alzheimer's Research & Therapy. 2015;7(1):5. DOI: 10.1186/s13195-014-0081-2

[127] Jacobsen FM, Comas-Díaz L. Donepezil for psychotropic-induced memory loss. The Journal of Clinical Psychiatry. 1999;**60**(10):698-704. PMID: 10549687

[128] Broad J, Kung V, Boundouki G, Aziz Q, De Maeyer J, Knowles C, et al. Cholinergic interactions between donepezil and prucalopride in human colon: Potential to treat severe intestinal dysmotility. British Journal of

Pharmacology. 2013;**170**(6):1253-1261. DOI: 10.1111/bph.12397

[129] Davidsson P, Blennow K, Andreasen N, Eriksson B, Minthon L, Hesse C. Differential increase in cerebrospinal fluid-acetylcholinesterase after treatment with acetylcholinesterase inhibitors in patients with Alzheimer's disease. Neuroscience Letters. 2001;**300**(3):157-160. PMID: 11226635

[130] Wilkinson DG, Francis PT, Schwam E, Payne-Parrish J. Cholinesterase inhibitors used in the treatment of Alzheimer's disease: The relationship between pharmacological effects and clinical efficacy. Drugs & Aging. 2004;**21**(7):453-478. PMID: 15132713

[131] Di Angelantonio S, Bernardi G, Mercuri NB. Donepezil modulates nicotinic receptors of substantia nigra dopaminergic neurons. British Journal of Pharmacology. 2004;**141**(4):644-652. DOI: 10.1038/sj.bjp.0705660

[132] Galvin J. The quick dementia rating system (QDRS): A rapid dementia staging tool. Alzheimer's & Dementia: Diagnosis, Assessment & Disease Monitoring. 2015;**1**(2):249-259. DOI: 10.1016/j.dadm.2015.03.003

[133] Galvin J. Improving the clinical detection of Lewy body dementia with the Lewy body composite risk score. Alzheimer's & Dementia: Diagnosis, Assessment & Disease Monitoring. 2015;**1**(3):316-324. DOI: 10.1016/j.dadm.2015.05.004

[134] Chew ML, Mulsant BH, Pollock BG, Lehman ME, Greenspan A, Mahmoud RA, et al. Anticholinergic activity of 107 medications commonly used by older adults. Journal of the American Geriatrics Society. 2008;**56**(7):1333-1341. DOI: 10.1111/j.1532-5415.2008.01737.x

[135] Lepkowsky CM. Donepezil for Lewy body constipation: A six month follow-up. Journal of Molecular and Genetic Medicine. 2017;**11**(3). DOI: 10.4172/1747-0862.1000287

[136] Lepkowsky CM. Donepezil for constipation in Lewy body disease: A twelve month follow-up. Journal of Molecular and Genetic Medicine. 2018;**12**(1). DOI: 10.4172/1747-0862.1000337

[137] Lepkowsky CM. Donepezil for α-synuclein constipation: An 18 month follow-up. POJ Clinical Case Reports. 2018;**1**(1):1-4. Available from: https://proskolar.org/wp-content/uploads/2018/08/Donepezil-for-%CE%B1%E2%80%90synuclein-Constipation-An-18-Month-Follow-Up.pdf [Accessed 08/02/2018]

Chapter 4

Imaging of Constipation and Its Complications

Alexander S. Somwaru

Abstract

Radiology is an important tool in the diagnosis and treatment of patients with constipation. Imaging provides both vital anatomic and functional information that may facilitate arriving at an accurate diagnosis, assessing for serious complications, and delivering the appropriate therapy in a timely fashion. In this chapter, we discuss how each imaging modality is used to image patients with constipation. Within this discussion, we review what information is provided by each modality and we detail complete imaging protocols and technical parameters for each test. Finally, we highlight key findings with illustrative images from radiography, fluoroscopy, CT, and MR imaging.

Keywords: imaging, radiology, stercoral colitis, computed tomography, CT, magnetic resonance imaging, MRI

1. Introduction

Radiology plays a pivotal role in the detection of constipation, identification of underlying etiologies, and revealing associated complications. Imaging evaluation of constipation has evolved from radiography and contrast enemas to advanced cross-sectional and functional imaging. A dilemma that physicians of medical and surgical specialties encounter when confronted with a patient with constipation is the decision of if or when radiology is indicated. The clinical presentation of the patient and what information is desired will ultimately govern if imaging is warranted and then what is the most appropriate exam to order. If the patient presents in the acute setting with a potential surgical emergency, fast and widely available imaging exams, such as radiography or computed tomography (CT), are the most appropriate exams to order. If the patient has a chronic issue or data regarding colorectal function is desired, a colorectal transit time exam with Sitz markers or defecography with fluoroscopy or magnetic resonance (MR) imaging are the exams of choice. With a diverse range of anatomic and functional imaging tests available, radiology has developed into an invaluable mechanism in the assessment of patients with constipation.

2. Radiography

Radiography, also known as plain film or X-ray, is a widely available, inexpensive, and easily obtained imaging test to assess for constipation. While the reported diagnostic sensitivity of radiography for the detection of constipation is 84%, the reported specificity is 72% [1]. Despite its relatively low sensitivity and specificity, radiographs serve as a basis for triage for further imaging work-up and assist in the therapeutic decision-making process. Inherent pitfalls in radiography of patients whom are constipated are other causes of colonic dilation, particularly adynamic ileus and colonic pseudo-obstruction [1].

Radiography is commonly used to image pediatric patients with constipation, particularly in the acute setting. However there is a unified consensus throughout the medical community to reduce non-essential and unnecessary radiation exposure to the pediatric population [2]. The latest consensus guidelines from the North American and European Societies of Pediatric Gastroenterology, Hepatology, and Nutrition advocate that constipation should be diagnosed clinically in pediatric patients because there is no reliable system to diagnose constipation and, instead, this modality may lead to misdiagnosis of more acute pathology [2]. Expert consensus also advocates that radiography has no role in imaging of children with functional constipation, which is best diagnosed with careful clinical assessment and physical examination [2].

2.1 Radiography technique

Anteroposterior (AP) images of the abdomen and pelvis in the supine position are performed to visualize and qualify the burden of feces, visualize the size of the colon, and assess for colonic obstruction. Erect and lateral decubitus images of the abdomen and pelvis to may be added if there is concern for complications of constipation such as free air from a perforation [1].

2.2 Key findings on radiography

The key radiographic findings of constipation are the presence of large fecal burden throughout the colon, luminal fecalomas, and a relative paucity or absence of luminal gas [3]. Feces appear as soft tissue opacities with internal mottled air (**Figures 1** and 2) [3].

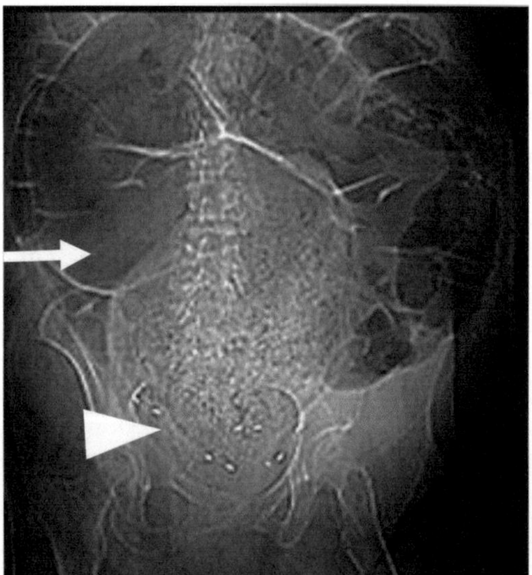

Figure 1.
AP radiograph of the abdomen and pelvis in a patient with constipation displays diffuse dilation of the colon (arrow) with an abrupt transition in luminal caliber by a large soft tissue opacity, which contains internal mottled air, indicative of feces (arrowhead).

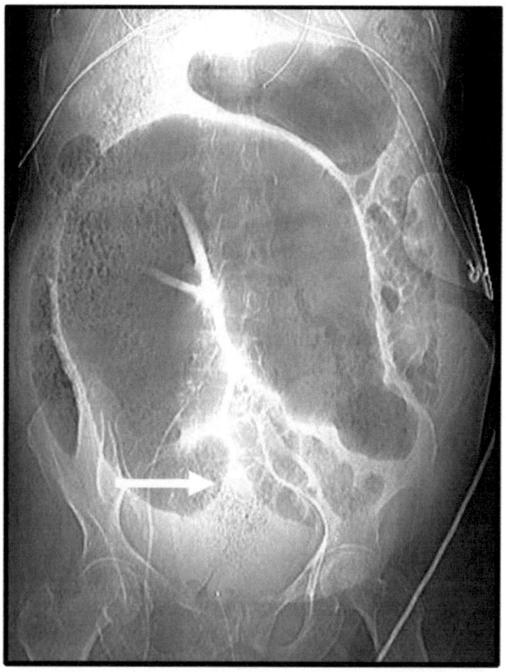

Figure 2.
AP radiograph of the abdomen and pelvis of patient with constipation shows a dilated colon with a transition in caliber due to a soft tissue opacity, which contains internal mottled air, characteristic of feces (arrow).

Radiography is helpful to assess for the presence of complications associated with constipation. Non-dependent images of the abdomen in the upright or left lateral decubitus positions may also be used for assessment of free air [1]. Bowel ischemia and infarction may be manifested on radiographs as pneumatosis, or air within the bowel wall, and/or portal venous gas, which projects over the silhouette of the liver [1]. Pneumoperitoneum from bowel perforation can be detected on radiography by air external to the bowel wall, air along the peritoneal ligaments, and air in the right upper abdominal quadrant [1]. If a surgical emergency is suspected on radiography, emergent surgical consultation is recommended. However, if surgery is not imminently planned or other treatment options are being considered, assessment of the severity and cause of the constipation with cross-sectional imaging becomes a priority. CT is the preferred imaging modality because of its superior sensitivity and specificity and it can potentially modify treatment.

Two entities that mimic mechanical causes of constipation are adynamic paralytic ileus and acute colonic pseudo-obstruction. Adynamic paralytic ileus is commonly due to medications, metabolic abnormalities, and recent surgery. Acute colonic pseudo-obstruction, also known as Ogilvie's Syndrome, is due to altered autonomic innervation of the colon and may also be caused by medications and metabolic disturbances [1].

Assessment of the small bowel and colon in pediatric patients may be challenging because the appearances, fold pattern, and location of the small bowel and colon overlap more so than in adult patients. There is also no established system to diagnose constipation in pediatric patients. Therefore radiography may be misleading in the assessment of pediatric patients it may result in missed diagnoses; this modality should be used in children in a limited fashion.

2.3 Radiography for colonic transit time: Sitz marker exam

A radiographic test that is used to estimate transit time of the colon is a Sitz marker exam [4]. In patients with constipation, this study may help discriminate between delayed colonic transit and defecation disorders.

2.3.1 Sitz marker exam

Patients are instructed to discontinue laxatives or any pro-motility medications. Otherwise no preparation is needed. The most common technique used is the ingestion of 20 or 24 Sitz markers in a single dose with a meal. Sitz markers are

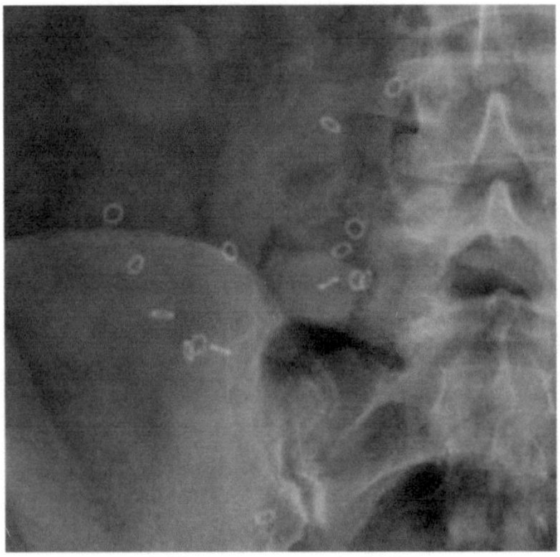

Figure 3.
Magnified AP radiograph of the pelvis shows Sitz markers.

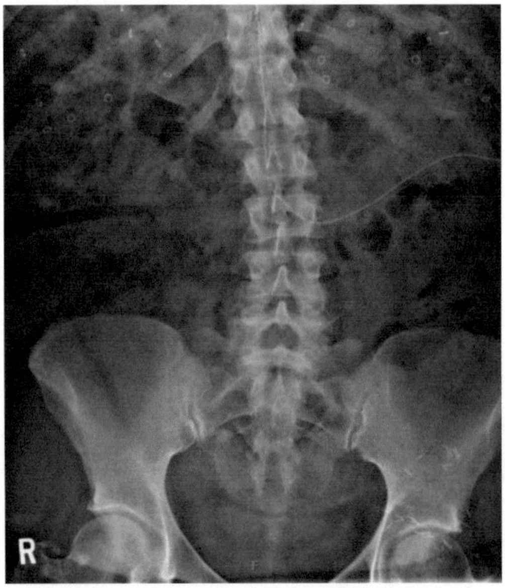

Figure 4.
AP radiograph of the abdomen and pelvis in this patient on day 3 of a Sitz marker exam, 18 of 20 Sitz markers are present and indicate that colonic transit will be delayed at 5 days.

Day	Sitz markers
1	≤16
2	≤8
3	≤4
4	≤2
5	≤1

Table 1.
Anticipated schedule of the number of retained Sitz markers on serial daily abdominal radiographs in a 20 Sitz marker exam. Day number is in the left column and retained Sitz marker number is in the right column.

small, plastic rings that contain radio-opaque material so they may be visible on radiographs (**Figure 3**) [4]. Then serial anteroposterior radiographic images of the abdomen and pelvis are obtained to monitor the clearance of the Sitz markers from the colon (**Figure 4**). A normal colonic transit time ranges between 24 and 56 h. Most patients will clear all of the Sitz markers in 4–5 days [4].

2.3.2 Key findings on Sitz marker exam

A normal colonic transit time, which is between 24 and 56 hours, corresponds to retention of less than 20% of the original Sitz markers at 5 days [4]. In a Sitz marker exam that used 20 Sitz markers, the anticipated schedule of the number of retained Sitz markers on serial daily abdominal radiographs is as follows (**Table 1**).

3. Fluoroscopy

Fluoroscopy employs the administration of contrast with real-time, moving radiographs to image both anatomy and function. Two fluoroscopic imaging techniques used to evaluate patients with constipation are contrast enema and evacuation proctography exams.

3.1 Contrast enema

Contrast enema may be valuable in the initial imaging assessment of patients with constipation because of it allows delineation of mechanical causes of constipation by displaying the luminal size of the colon and rectum, site(s) of transition in luminal caliber, and the length of involvement [5]. This exam is unique because it may be both diagnostic and therapeutic: the instillation of contrast material into the colon and rectum may relieve fecal impaction [5].

3.1.1 Contrast enema technique

Prior to the exam, patients undergo a bowel cleanse preparation with an oral laxative, such as magnesium citrate or polyethylene glycol. Contrast enema exams are performed with fluoroscopy and may be performed with either single contrast: barium or water-soluble contrast only or double contrast: barium or water-soluble contrast with the insufflation of air or carbon dioxide.

Pre-procedural radiographic anteroposterior images of the abdomen and pelvis and a left lateral radiographic view of pelvis are obtained. The patient then lies in the left lateral decubitus position on the fluoroscopy table. A digital rectal exam in performed. Then a thin, small-gauge, flexible catheter is placed into the rectum. This catheter is typically paired with a small, balloon that is inflated to ensure that the catheter does not back out of the rectum. If double contrast is performed, air or carbon dioxide is gently insufflated by hand pump to patient tolerance. The contrast is then instilled into the rectum and colon by gravity. During contrast administration, fluoroscopic-guided spot radiographic left and right lateral and left and right posterior oblique images of the rectum, rectosigmoid junction, sigmoid colon, descending colon and splenic flexure are obtained. Then an anteroposterior view of the transverse colon and a left posterior oblique view of hepatic flexure are obtained. Finally anteroposterior and posterior oblique images of the ascending colon, cecum, ileocecal valve, and the terminal ileum, are obtained. At the end of the exam, the contrast is emptied out of the colon by gravity and a post evacuation anteroposterior radiographic view of the abdomen and pelvis is obtained.

3.1.2 Key findings on contrast enema

Contrast enema exams can depict filling defects in the colon and rectum from feces and fecalomas from constipation or an obstructive mass, such as malignancy (**Figure 5**) [5].

Colonic and rectal luminal size and the presence, degree, and length of strictures are all displayed and can be assessed on contrast enemas [5, 6]. Strictures, which are due to fibrosis from repeated inflammation or de-vascularization, may be caused by diverticulitis (**Figure 6**), ischemia, prior radiation or surgery (**Figure 7**), and inflammatory bowel disease (**Figure 8**) [5, 6].

Contrast enema is a dynamic imaging modality in the assessment of pediatric patients with constipation [7]. Contrast enemas are invaluable in both the diagnosis and extent of involvement for Hirschsprung's disease, an entity that results in constipation due aganglionosis, or absence of the ganglion cells, in the distal colon and rectum [7]. The denervated distal colon or rectum is small in luminal size with proximal dilation [7]. Early filling views of the sigmoid colon and rectum allow for detection of an abnormal sigmoid colon to rectum size ratio and fasciculation or saw-tooth irregularity of the denervated segment [7].

While contrast enema can reliably display these causes of constipation, computed tomography (CT) may characterize these entities with greater spatial and

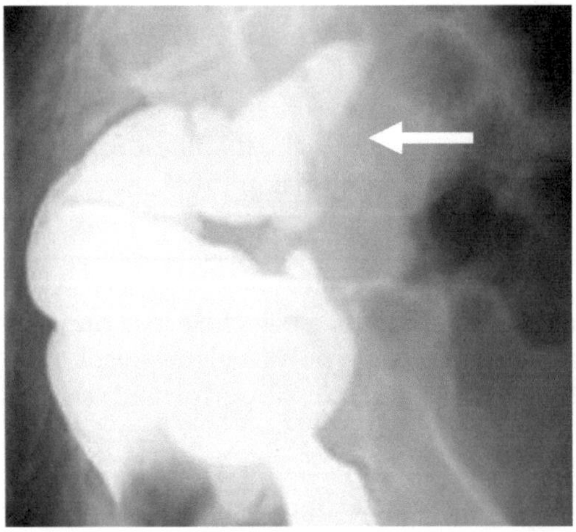

Figure 5.
Contrast enema image of the sigmoid colon in a patient with constipation and irregular bowel movements shows an abrupt transition (arrow) with obstruction of passage of contrast. The patient was referred for a colonoscopy and then surgery for resection of an adenocarcinoma.

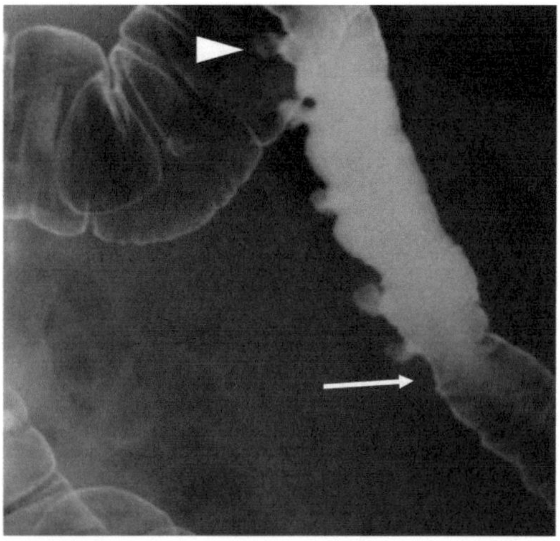

Figure 6.
A patient with abnormal and irregular bowel movements and constipation following an episode of acute diverticulitis underwent a contrast enema. Adjacent to multiple diverticula (arrowhead) in the descending colon, there is focal, short-segment, low-grade stricture (arrow) from prior diverticulitis.

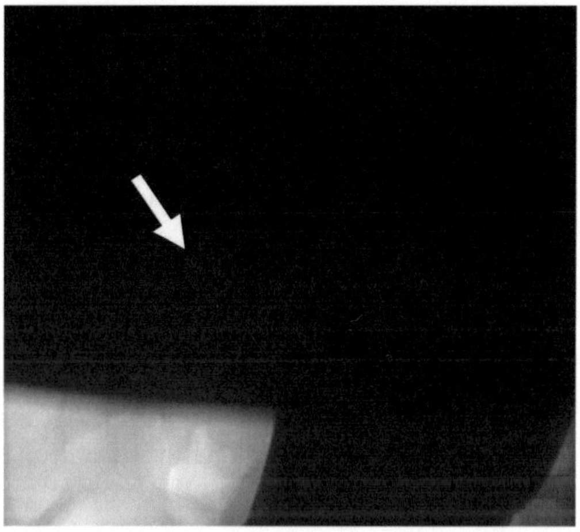

Figure 7.
Contrast enema image of a patient with constipation and decreased bowel movements; she has a history of cervical cancer that was treated with radiation therapy. There is a short-segment, high-grade stricture (arrow) in the sigmoid colon due to prior radiation therapy.

temporal resolution, in a shorter time, with improved patient comfort, and that is more available, particularly in the emergent setting [8]. CT also permits visualization of extra-colorectal structures [8]. Therefore these causes of constipation are discussed in further depth in the CT section of this chapter.

3.2 Fluoroscopic defecography

Defecography is a fluoroscopic exam that provides valuable data for patients with constipation that is caused by both anatomic and functional disorders, which range from pelvic floor dysfunction to spastic pelvic floor syndrome. This exam is typically performed in adult and adolescent patients whom may follow instructions for the dynamic portion of the exam.

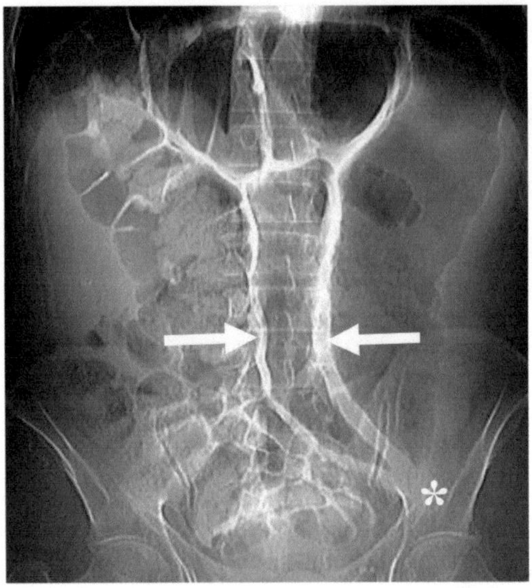

Figure 8.
A patient with ulcerative colitis underwent a contrast enema. AP image after evacuation of contrast shows contrast outlining diffuse colonic wall thickening (arrows) and dilatation with smooth tapering in the sigmoid colon (asterisk).

3.2.1 Fluoroscopic defecography technique

Pre-procedural bowel preparation consists of a bowel cleanse preparation with an oral laxative, such as magnesium citrate or polyethylene glycol. Barium may be administered in the vagina (5 mL barium instillation) and small bowel (500 mL barium oral ingestion) to simultaneously assess these structures in relation to the colon and rectum.

The patient is placed on the fluoroscopy table in left lateral decubitus position. 120–240 mL of barium paste is introduced into the rectum with a large-bore, soft catheter. Then spot lateral radiographic images of the patient at rest in the left lateral decubitus position with knees flexed to recreate the seated position. The patient is then positioned in a special defecography chair. Continuous and spot right lateral images of the seated patient are obtained at rest at rest, during strain (Valsalva maneuver), and then during defecation. A post-evacuation image during strain is obtained to assess for retained barium paste.

3.2.2 Key findings on fluoroscopic defecography

Defecography is a highly sensitive modality for the detection and classification of rectocele and rectal prolapse [9, 10]. A rectocele is the abnormal bulging or protrusion of the rectal wall due to a fascial or ligamentous defect [10]. A rectocele may cause inhibit defecation due to weakening of the vector force during strain [9, 10]. Feces may become entrapped in rectoceles that in turn results in incomplete evacuation [9, 10]. The presence of an anterior rectocele (**Figure 9**) is indicative of a defect in the recto-vaginal fascia whereas the presence of a posterior rectocele indicates a defect in the anococcygeal ligament [9, 10]. Rectal prolapse may cause constipation by infolding of the rectum that is caused by repetitive straining and fascial disruption [9, 10].

Rectoceles are measured and classified on the basis of distance of the anterior or posterior rectal wall from the anal canal axis [9, 11, 12]. Rectal prolapses are classified by mucosa-only or full wall-thickness involvement and intra-rectal, internal

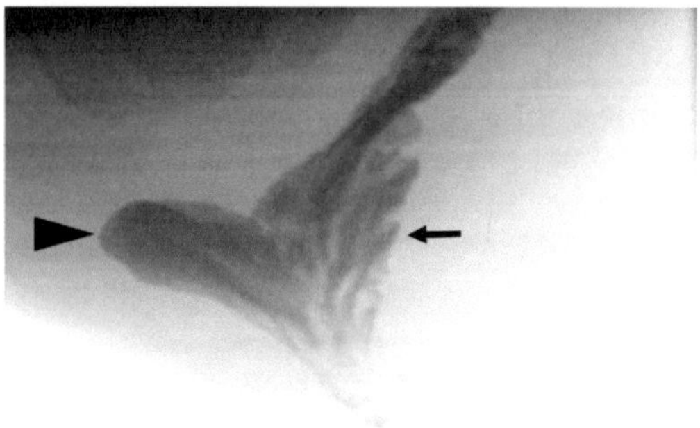

Figure 9.
Evacuation image from a fluoroscopic defecography in a patient with difficult evacuation and constipation shows a mucosal, intra-rectal prolapse (arrow) and an anterior rectocele (arrowhead), which incompletely empties.

intra-anal, or external location (**Figure 9**) [9, 11, 12]. While fluoroscopic defecography has been shown to be highly sensitive for rectal prolapse detection, MR defecography allows for similarly reliable and accurate classification of rectocele and rectal prolapse type due to superior tissue resolution [12].

4. Magnetic resonance (MR) defecography

As an analogue to fluoroscopic defecography, MR defecography plays a vital role in the management of patients with constipation that is caused by both anatomic and functional disorders, which range from pelvic floor dysfunction to spastic pelvic floor syndrome [9, 11, 12]. High resolution and dynamic MR techniques provide detailed anatomic and physiologic information of the colon, rectum, and pelvic floor [9, 11, 12]. This data may then be used to discriminate patients that need surgery from those that need more conservative therapy [9, 11, 12]. For example, many patients with rectoceles from pelvic floor dysfunction will never improve without surgical repair whereas patients with functional constipation are treated with positive biologic feedback [9, 11, 12].

MR defecography is typically performed in adult and adolescent patients whom may tolerate confined space of the bore of the magnet and follow instructions for the dynamic portion of the exam. Challenges to MR imaging are pre-procedural preparation and scan times that are longer than radiography or CT exams. Also MR imaging exams may be limited in certain patients because of claustrophobia, as well as medical devices and orthopedic metallic hardware.

4.1 MR defecography technique

Prior to the exam, patients undergo a bowel cleanse preparation with an oral laxative, such as magnesium citrate or polyethylene glycol, and fast for 6 h. The patient is instructed to use one rectal enema the night before the examination and another up to 1 h before the exam. The patient lies in the right decubitus position on an absorbent, waterproof pad on the MR table and approximately 100–150 mL of warmed ultrasound gel is instilled in the rectum with a flexible tube. In female patients, 60 mL of ultrasound gel may be instilled into the vagina for to simultaneously assess the vagina and cervix in relation to the colon and rectum.

Simple and clear communication is important to establish with the patient during the examination to ensure direct instructions are followed that will in turn yield the best possible images. A phased-array torso coil is used to acquire sagittal, coronal, and axial T2-weighted steady-state fast spin echo (SSFSE) MR images: 24–30 cm field of view (FOV), 6 mm thickness, 512 × 256 matrix, repetition time (TR) = 5170 ms, echo time (TE) = 137 ms, from the superior border of the pubic symphysis to the lower end of the anal canal. Are then obtained of the entire pelvis. T2-weighted MR images are helpful in assessing for wall edema or masses and accentuate mucosal features against a bright background created by rectal ultrasound gel contrast. The high-resolution images provide superb soft tissue detail for hernias and muscular or fascial defects.

Dynamic fast imaging employing steady-state acquisition is then performed. The FOV is centered at the rectum and then imaging is performed at rest, during strain (Valsalva maneuver), and then during defecation. Serial, single-section mid-sagittal SSFSE MR images (30 cm FOV, 8 mm thickness, 256 × 256 matrix, TR = 3840 ms, TE = 1670 ms) are acquired every 2 s and repeated 15–20 times and viewed as a cine loop. Gradient echo imaging may also be used for the dynamic sequences. Imaging is also performed of the patient while performing squeeze maneuver to evaluate puborectalis muscle contraction. The use of these dynamic sequences allows real-time functional imaging.

4.2 Key findings on MR defecography

The excellent tissue resolution of MR imaging provides valuable information on anatomic abnormalities of the rectum and pelvic floor. The dynamic component of MR imaging enables assessment of function and physiology. MR imaging has a high sensitivity of the presence of rectoceles (**Figure 10**) and rectal prolapse (**Figure 10**) [9, 11]. Rectoceles are measured and classified on the basis of distance of the anterior or posterior rectal wall from the anal canal axis [9, 11]. A bulge of the rectum that measures less than 2 cm is normal; over 2 cm is abnormal and diagnostic of a rectocele [9, 11, 12]. Rectoceles that protrude up to 3 cm from the normal margin are a significant cause of constipation or incomplete defecation [9, 11, 12]. A rectocele of more than 4 cm is classified as large [9, 11, 12].

Rectal prolapse may cause constipation due to rectal wall infolding that is induced by chronic straining and fascial disruption [9, 11, 12]. Rectal prolapse can only involve the mucosa or the entire wall thickness [9, 11, 12]. Rectal prolapses

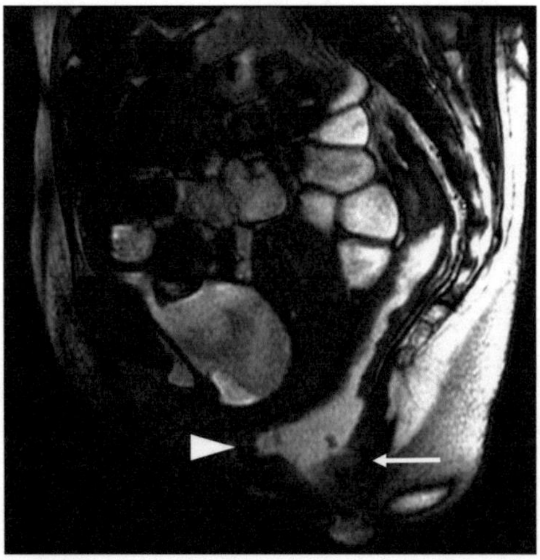

Figure 10.
Mid-sagittal SSFSE MR image of the pelvis during evacuation in a patient with constipation shows a large anterior rectocele (arrowhead) and internal intra-rectal prolapse (arrow).

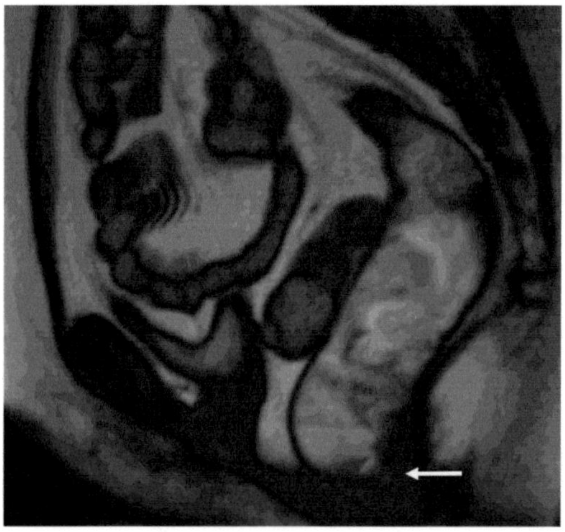

Figure 11.
Mid-sagittal gradient echo MR image of the pelvis during evacuation in a patient with chronic constipation show persistent puborectalis muscular contraction (arrow) without expulsion of intra-rectal gel.

may also be internal intra-rectal, internal intra-anal, or external [9, 11, 12]. Although fluoroscopy has been shown to be a highly sensitive modality for the detection of rectal prolapse relative to MR imaging, the superior resolution of MR imaging similarly provides accurate differentiation of mucosa-only prolapse from full-wall-thickness prolapse [9, 11, 12]. Thus MR imaging provides crucial anatomical and functional information for surgical planning and enables accurate discrimination between the subtypes of rectal prolapse [9, 11, 12].

Spastic pelvic floor syndrome, or anismus, is caused by paradoxical and involuntary contraction of the puborectalis muscle in the pelvic floor [9, 11]. It results in non-relaxation of the external anal sphincter complex and impairs normal defecation [9, 11]. This causes constipation with prolonged and incomplete defecation [9, 11]. Imaging findings include persistent puborectalis muscular contraction during the strain (Valsalva maneuver) and defecation phases, absence of pelvic floor descent, and an abnormally acute anorectal angle (**Figure 11**) [9, 11].

5. Computed tomography (CT)

CT is the most important imaging modality in the evaluation of patients with known or suspected constipation. It is readily available, performed quickly, allows assessment for potential complications, and permits visualization of extra-colonic structures. The advent of multi-detector CT scanners with improved technical protocols has resulted in faster and more available imaging, particularly in the acute setting. Multi-planar and thin section reconstruction capability may allow for identification of sites of obstruction in the colon and rectum and delineation of colorectal morphology. CT has a reported sensitivity of 96% and specificity of 93% in the identification of constipation. Additional benefits of CT are visualization of complications associated with constipation, particularly stercoral colitis, ischemia, and perforation, and other organ systems for comorbid conditions that may cause constipation [1, 3, 13–15]. CT is widely used to image adult patients however it is used judiciously in pediatric patients to avoid radiation exposure. If, however, a pediatric patient has constipation that may be secondarily caused by another acute pathology, CT can be of vital importance to diagnosis and management. Radiation dose reduction and modulation may be performed to reduced exposure to pediatric patients.

5.1 CT technique

CT has been particularly valuable in the determination of which patients would benefit from conservative medical management or immediate surgical intervention. CT imaging is typically performed using a 64 or 128-section multi-detector row scanner. Each exam is acquired during a single breath hold and in helical mode. Typical exposure settings are 120 kVp, automated tube current modulation with minimum tube current 100–150 mAs and beam pitch, 0.8–1.375. The administration of intravenous (IV) non-ionic contrast material is advised to assess for the presence of a colonic mass, or wall ischemia or inflammation. Exposure settings are set to 100 kVp and automated tube current modulation with minimum tube current is reduced to 80–100 mAs. If IV contrast is administered (contrast-enhanced), a single-phase technique is used with the acquisition of portal venous phase images 70 s after the IV administration of nonionic contrast material that is injected at a rate of 3–5 mL/s. Positive oral contrast material may or may not be used, depending on the indication and urgency or timing of the exam. Multi-planar reconstruction imaging in the coronal and sagittal planes, which are automatically created at the CT technologist's console, is routinely used. These images may be of great value in not only the diagnosis of constipation but also in the detection of the variety of common and uncommon causes and potential complications.

5.2 Key findings on CT

CT may have a substantial and significant impact on the clinical management of the patient by helping to answer major questions: is the patient constipated? Do feces

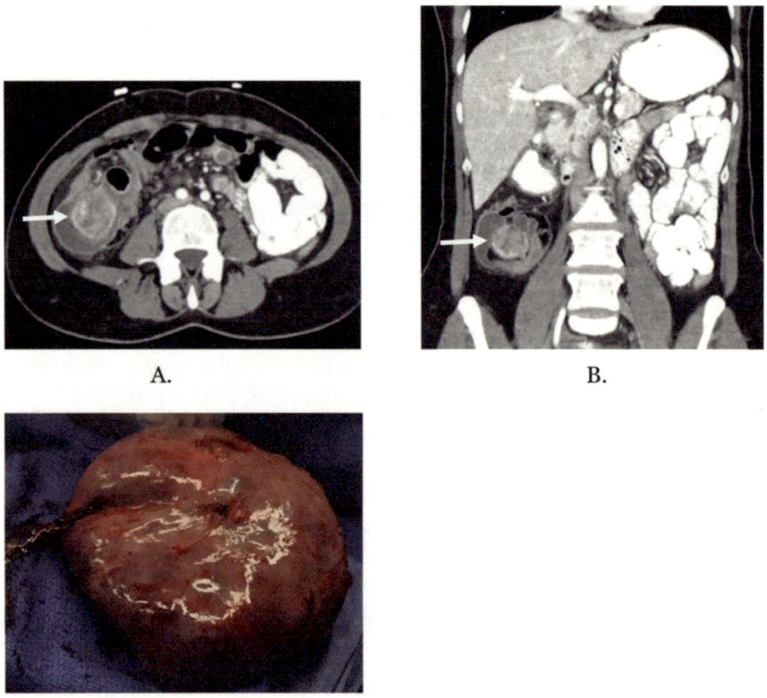

C.

Figure 12.
(A and B) Axial and coronal images from a contrast-enhanced CT of the abdomen and pelvis of a patient with constipation and bloody bowel movements. There is an enhancing polypoid mass that arises in the cecum and extends into the lumen. (C) The patient then underwent colonoscopy and right colectomy for resection of a colonic adenocarcinoma.

impact the rectum? Are there associated complications of constipation, such as stercoral colitis, ischemia, or perforation? Is the colon obstructed? If the colon is obstructed, can the cause of the constipation be identified, as well as its exact site? CT is particularly useful in the detection of the variety of mechanical causes of constipation.

5.2.1 Malignancy

Primary colonic malignancy is one of the most common mechanical causes [1]. Colonic malignancy is shown on CT as an annular, semi-annular, polypoid, or ulcerated mass that arises from the colon and extends into the lumen or through the wall (**Figure 12A–C**) [16].

5.2.2 Strictures

Strictures are another mechanical cause of constipation. The pathophysiological mechanism for the development of a stricture is fibrosis from repeated inflammation or de-vascularization [17]. The main causes of strictures are diverticulitis, ischemia, inflammatory bowel disease, and prior medical therapy like surgery or radiation [17]. CT may display ancillary features of the primary cause of the stricture that may lead to an accurate diagnosis [17]. If the patient has colonic diverticular disease, repeated episodes of diverticulitis may cause a stricture (**Figure 13**) [15, 18].

Multiple and prolonged episodes of inflammation Crohn disease and ulcerative colitis are types of inflammatory bowel disease that may cause a fixed stricture (**Figure 14**) [15, 19]. Surgical and treatment history may reveal that the fixed stenosis is likely due to adhesive fibrosis from a surgical anastomosis or (**Figure 15A** and **B**) [15].

5.2.3 Stercoral colitis

CT plays an invaluable role in the detection of a significant and even fatal complication of constipation that is known as stercoral colitis. Elderly patients,

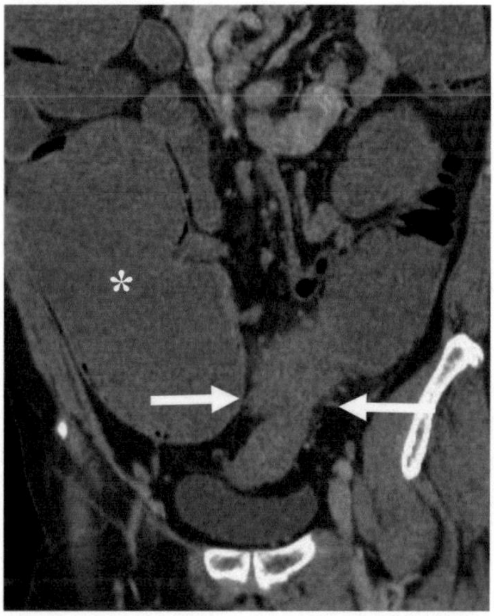

Figure 13.
A patient with several prior episodes of diverticulitis presented with pain and constipation. Coronal image from a contrast-enhanced CT shows a significant amount of feces and fluid in the dilated colon (asterisk) due to sigmoid colonic wall thickening and pericolonic fat stranding in the setting of diverticulosis, compatible with a diverticular stricture.

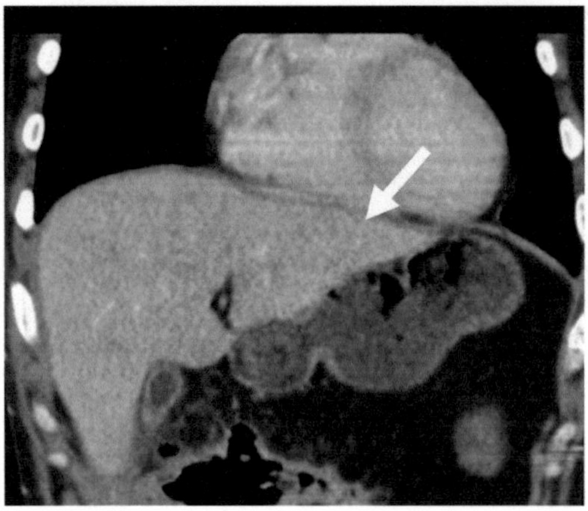

Figure 14.
Coronal image from a contrast-enhanced CT of a patient with Crohn disease displays a short-segment stricture in the mid-transverse colon (arrow) that results in a short-segment stricture (arrowhead) and upstream constipation.

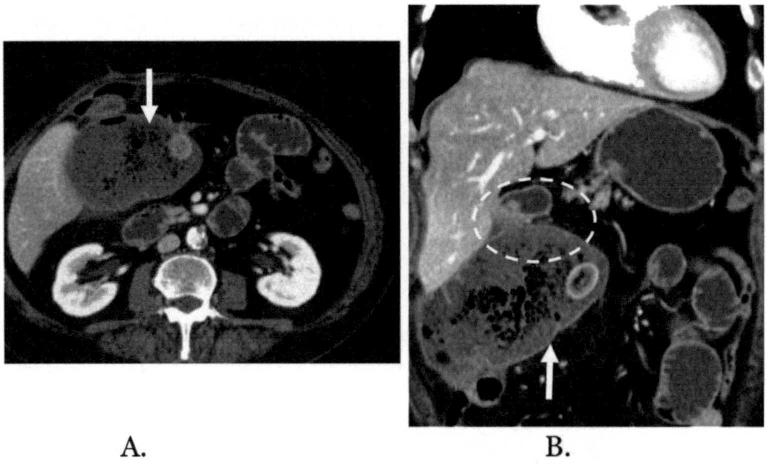

Figure 15.
(A and B) A patient presented with severe constipation and no bowel movements for over 1 week. Axial and coronal images from a contrast-enhanced CT show large feces that distend the cecum and ascending colon (arrow) due to a stricture at the hepatic flexure (circle). The stricture is due to post-surgical fibrosis that developed between the colon and the site of a prior cholecystectomy (circle).

especially those with chronic diseases, are at the highest risk for development of stercoral colitis [3, 13–15]. Signs and symptoms of stercoral colitis are not specific; however, the most common complaints are constipation and pain [3, 13, 14]. Serologic tests and physical examination are also not specific [3, 13, 14].

The pathophysiology of stercoral colitis begins with constipation. Chronic constipation, without treatment or intervention, may lead to fecal impaction and fecaloma formation [3, 13, 14, 20]. A fecaloma is dehydrated, compacted feces. Impacted feces and fecalomas exert pressure upon the walls of the colon and rectum that in turn impairs vascular perfusion [3, 13, 14, 20]. Hypoperfusion leads to ischemia, infarction, and necrosis of the colon and rectum with consequent perforation [3, 13, 14]. The sigmoid colon is the most common site because: (1) it is the narrowest point in the colon, thereby impeding the transit of dehydrated feces and (2) the rectosigmoid vascular watershed region, known as Sudeck's point, is susceptible to ischemia [3, 13, 14].

DOI: http://dx.doi.org/10.5772/intechopen.81472

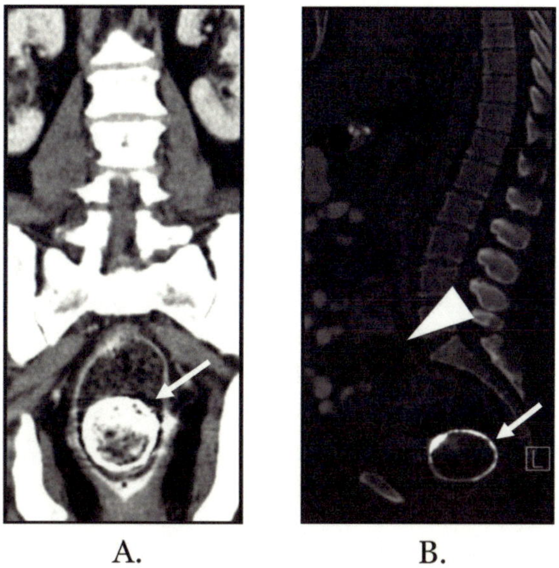

Figure 16.
(A and B) Coronal and sagittal contrast-enhanced CT images of a patient with constipation show fecal impaction in a dilated colon and rectum (arrowhead) with a large, rim-calcified fecaloma (arrow) that causes stercoral colitis.

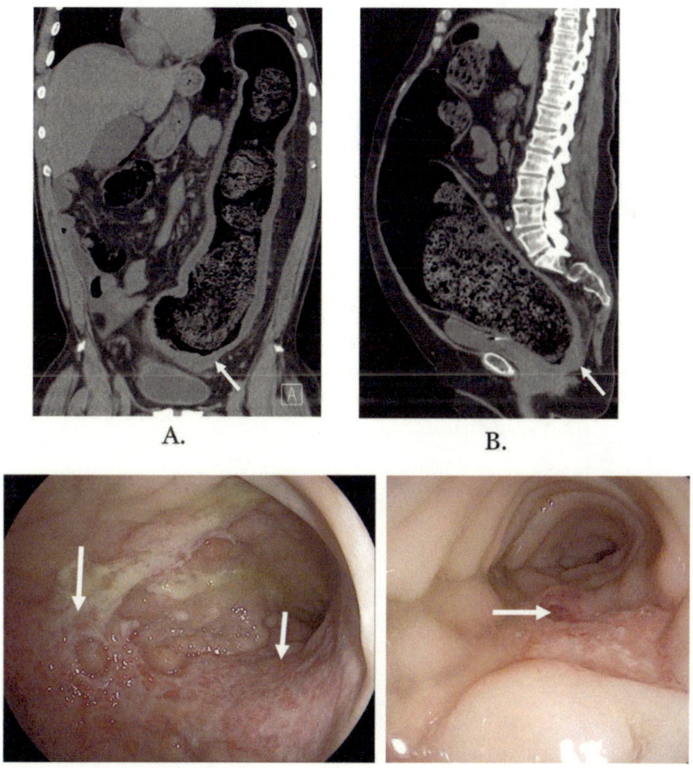

Figure 17.
(A and B) Sagittal and axial non-contrast CT images of a patient with severe abdominal distention and constipation show a dilated colon with a large volume of feces and concentric wall thickening (arrows), indicative of stercoral colitis. (C and D) The majority of the fecaloma was removed in a piecemeal fashion with irrigation and retrieval devices. Images from the colonoscopy show friable, dusky, and erythematous mucosa (arrows), consistent with stercoral colitis and ischemia.

Radiography can detect fecal impaction and fecalomas in the colon and rectum however provides no sensitive or specific findings of stercoral colitis [3, 13, 14]. CT is diagnostic of stercoral colitis and its complications and can also exclude alternative causes of pain [3, 13–15]. The finding that is present in all patients with stercoral colitis is a fecaloma (**Figure 16A** and **B**) [3, 13–15]. Proximal to the fecaloma, the colon may or may not be dilated. The walls of the colon and rectum are asymmetrically thickened to greater than 0.3 cm and my have increased attenuation due to ischemic hemorrhage (**Figure 17A–D**) [3, 13, 14]. Extra-colorectal findings are inflammatory stranding of the fat that surrounds the colon and rectum and extra-luminal air, which is indicative of a perforation (**Figure 18A–C**) [3, 13]. Complications of stercoral colitis are perforation, abscess, peritonitis, sepsis, and death; mortality has been reported to approach nearly 50% [3, 13–15].

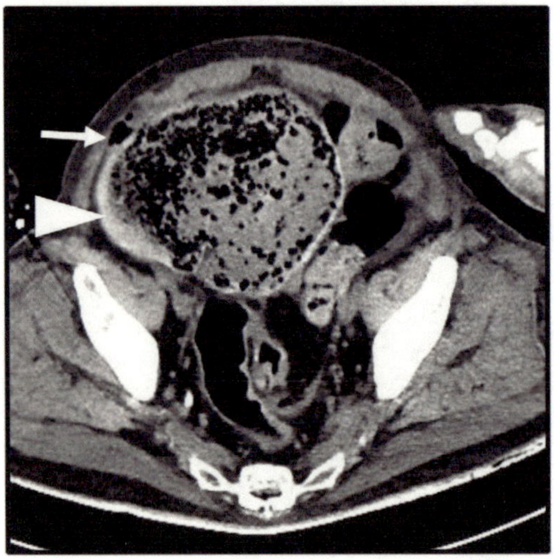

A.

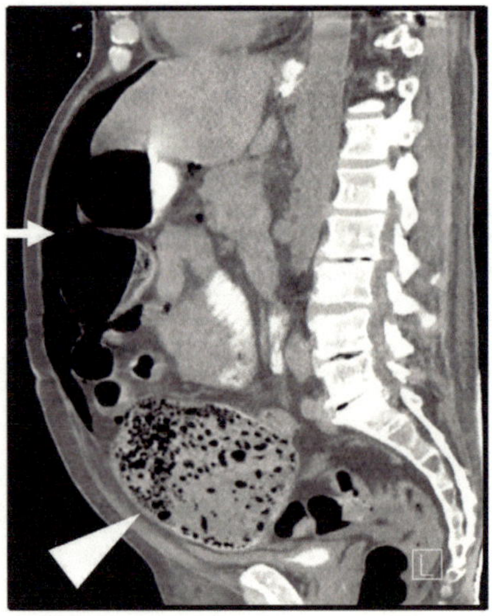

B.

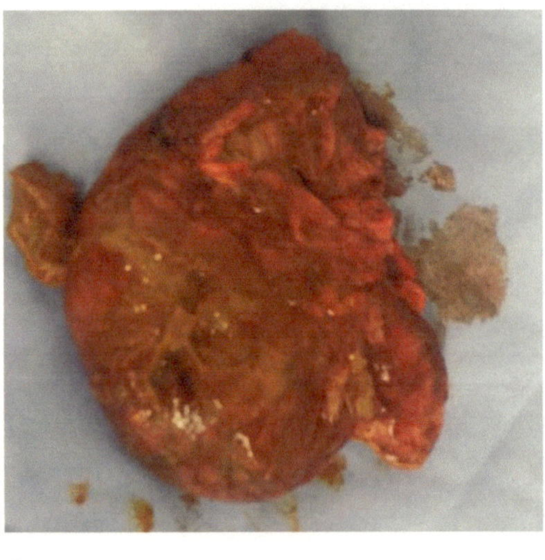

C.

Figure 18.
(A and B) Sagittal and axial contrast-enhanced CT images show fecal impaction of the cecum with asymmetric wall thickening (arrowheads) and extraluminal air (arrow) adjacent to a thinned segment of the cecal wall and throughout the peritoneum (arrow), consistent with a perforation. (C) Gross surgical specimen of the resected and perforated cecum, which is filled with feces.

6. Conclusions

The clinical presentation of a patient with constipation will help govern if imaging is warranted and what is the most appropriate exam to order. Identification of the specific etiologies and associated complications of constipation is facilitated by both anatomic and functional imaging which range from basic radiography to MR imaging. Understanding what information each imaging modality can provide is of paramount importance to order the appropriate test, make an accurate diagnosis, and guide the appropriate management.

Acknowledgements

The author acknowledges Shaile Philips, M.D. for her contributions and mentorship.

Conflict of interest

The author declares no conflict of interest.

Thanks

The author thanks his parents for their support and guidance.

Author details

Alexander S. Somwaru
Department of Radiology, Icahn School of Medicine at Mount Sinai, New York, USA

*Address all correspondence to: alexander.somwaru@mountsinai.org

References

[1] Jaffe T, Thompson W. Large bowel obstruction in the adult: Classic radiographic and CT findings, etiology, and mimics. Radiology. 2015;**275**(3):651-663

[2] Ferguson CC, Gray MP, Diaz M, Boyd KP. Reducing unnecessary imaging for patients with constipation in the pediatric emergency department. Pediatrics. 2017;**140**(1):e1-e7

[3] Saksonov M, Bachar GN, Morgenstern S, et al. Stercoral colitis: A lethal disease-computed tomographic findings and clinical characteristic. Journal of Computer Assisted Tomography. 2014;**38**(5):721-726

[4] Lin HC, Prather C, Fisher RS, et al. Measurement of gastrointestinal transit. Digestive Diseases and Sciences. 2005;**50**(6):989-1004

[5] Sawai RS. Management of colonic obstruction: A review. Clinics of Colon and Rectal Surgery. 2012;**25**(4):200-203

[6] Drozdz W, Budzynski P. Change in mechanical bowel obstruction demographic and etiological patterns during the past century: Observations from one health care institution. Archives of Surgery. 2012;**147**(2):175-180

[7] O'Donovan AN, Habra G, Somers S, et al. Diagnosis of Hirschsprung's disease. AJR: American Journal of Roentgenology. 1996;**167**(2):517-520

[8] Taourel P, Kessler N, Lesnik A, et al. Helical CT of large bowel obstruction. Abdominal Imaging. 2003;**28**(2):267-275

[9] Hassan HH, Elnekiedy AM, Elshazly WG, Naguib NN. Modified MR defecography without rectal filling in obstructed defecation syndrome: Initial experience. European Journal of Radiology. 2016;**85**(9):1673-1681

[10] Karasick S, Karasick D, Karasick SR. Functional disorders of the anus and rectum: Findings on defecography. AJR: American Journal of Roentgenology. 1993;**160**(4):777-782

[11] Colaiacomo MC, Masselli G, Polettini E, et al. Dynamic MR imaging of the pelvic floor: A pictorial review. Radiographics. 2009;**29**(3):e35

[12] Law YM, Fielding JR. MRI of pelvic floor dysfunction: Review. AJR: American Journal of Roentgenology. 2008;**191**(6 Suppl):S45-S53

[13] Wu CH, Wang LJ, Wong YC, et al. Necrotic stercoral colitis: Importance of computed tomography findings. World Journal of Gastroenterology. 2011;**17**(3):379-384

[14] Heffernan C, Pachter HL, Megibow AJ, Macari M. Stercoral colitis leading to fatal peritonitis: CT findings. AJR: American Journal of Roentgenology. 2005;**184**(4):1189-1193

[15] Somwaru AS, Philips S. Imaging of uncommon causes of large-bowel obstruction. AJR: American Journal of Roentgenology. 2017;**209**(5):W277-W286

[16] Filippone A, Ambrosini R, Fuschi M, et al. Preoperative T and N staging of colorectal cancer: Accuracy of contrast-enhanced multi-detector row CT colonography-initial experience. Radiology. 2004;**231**(1):83-90

[17] Cappell MS, Batke M. Mechanical obstruction of the small bowel and colon. Medical Clinics of North America. 2008;**92**(3):575-597

[18] Gryspeerdt S, Lefere P. Chronic diverticulitis vs. colorectal cancer: Findings on CT colonography. Abdominal Imaging. 2012;**37**(6):1101-1109

[19] Punwani S, Rodriguez-Justo M, Bainbridge A, et al. Mural inflammation in Crohn disease: Location-matched histologic validation of MR imaging features. Radiology. 2009;**252**(3):712-720

[20] Fagelman D, Warhit JM, Reiter JD, Geiss AC. CT diagnosis of fecaloma. Journal of Computer Assisted Tomography. 1984;**8**(3):559-561

Chapter 5

Therapeutic Role of Natural Products Containing Tannin for Treatment of Constipation

Dae Youn Hwang

Abstract

Many herbal plants and medicinal foods with laxative effects have been reported as novel therapeutic strategies for the treatment of constipation and its related diseases. Indeed, several natural products containing tannins exhibit remarkable laxative effects in a constipation model. Therefore, we reviewed the laxative effects and the mechanism of action of natural products containing tannins because tannins have a wide range of pharmacological activities against human diseases. These products improved the excretion parameters, histological structure, mucin secretion and the downstream signaling pathway of muscarinic acetylcholine receptors (mAChRs) in the constipation model. This review provides strong evidence that various medicinal plants containing tannins are important candidates for improving chronic constipation.

Keywords: laxative effects, tannin, natural products, excretion parameters, constipation

1. Introduction

Chronic constipation is a complex gastrointestinal disease that is characterized by infrequent bowel movements, difficult defecation, sensation of incomplete bowel evacuation, sensation of anorectal obstruction, and the need for excessive straining [1–3]. This disease can be roughly classified into three groups: (i) constipation in the elderly and cancer patients; (ii) constipation related to neuromuscular diseases and (iii) functional constipation [1]. Constipation can be caused by a variety of factors including insufficient dietary fiber or fluid intake, decreased physical activity, drug administration, colorectal cancer obstruction, and hypothyroidism [4].

Meanwhile, the most common types of drugs used to treat patients with chronic constipation can be classified into bulk laxatives, osmotic laxatives, emollient laxatives, and prokinetic and prosecretory agents [1, 5, 6]. Among these, stimulant laxatives such as bisacodyl and natrium picosulfate are commonly administered to chronic patients although they have some limitations including high costs and undesirable side effects [7]. These laxatives significantly enhance the motility and secretion of the intestine by regulating electrolyte transport by the intestinal mucosa [8]. Many bulking agents and osmotic laxatives successfully treat constipation in elderly and cancer patients and in neuromuscular diseases, while prokinetic and prosecretory agents are prescribed to patients with functional constipation (**Table 1**) [9].

Drug class	Generic name	Comments	Dose
Bulking agents	Psyllium Ispaghula	Effective Effective	25–30 g daily in divided doses 3.5 g to three times daily
Osmotic laxative	Polyethylene glycol	Effective Unpalatable taste	17 g in 237 ml solution daily
	Lactulose	Effective May causes bloating, flatulence and cramping	13–30 ml (667 mg/ml) daily
Stimulant laxatives	Bisacodyl	Effective, but the effects subside with time, can cause cramping	5–20 mg daily
	Natrium picosulfate		5–10 mg daily
Emollient laxative	Mineral oil	Effective	5–10 cm^3 daily
	Glycerin suppositories	Effective Initiates evacuation by distending the rectum	On demand
Prokinetic and prosecretory agents	Prucalopride	Effective. May cause headache, nausea, abdominal pain and diarrhea. These adverse events occur within the first 24 h of treatment and are short lived	2 mg daily
	Linaclotide	Diarrhea is the most common side effect	290 μg daily

Table 1.
Classification of drugs used to treat patients with chronic constipation [1].

To date, the laxative activities of natural products containing various bioactive compounds have been investigated in terms of the regulation of intestinal motility, ileum tension, frequency of defecation, and number of stools. Leaf extracts of *Aloe ferox* Mill., agarwood (*Aquilaria sinensis*, *A. crasna*), and common fig (*Ficus carica*) paste are reported to significantly increase the total stool weight and intestinal motility and to normalize body weight in constipated rats treated with loperamide (Lop) [10–12]. The water extract of Cactus (*Opuntia humifusa*) successfully improves the stool number and water content, as well as the histological parameters of the intestine [13]. High laxative activity and improvement of constipation symptoms were also observed after treatment with *Mareya micrantha* (Benth.) Mull. Arg. (Euphorbiaceae) in the Lop-induced constipation model [14]. A laxative effect compared to the standard drug (bisacodyl) was also detected with the methanol and hexane extracts of *Senna macranthera* leaves [15]. Furthermore, an aqueous extract of *Liriope platyphylla* recovered the frequency and weight of stools, villus length, crypt layer thickness, muscle thickness, mucin secretion, and accumulation of lipid droplets in crypt enterocytes [16]. The laxative effects of *L. platyphylla* correlated with the signaling pathway of mAChRs [16]. Although the laxative activity of many natural products has been reported, a relationship between natural products containing tannin and laxative effects has never been focused until now.

In the present review, we focused on the laxative effects and mechanism of action of natural products containing tannin in a constipation model. This study is the first to suggest that natural products containing tannin may be as effective at alleviating constipation as commercial drugs such as bisacodyl, sennoside calcium, and docusate sodium.

2. Laxative effects and mechanism of action of natural products containing tannin

2.1 Role of tannin as health-benefiting biomolecules

Tannins are the most abundant secondary metabolites in plants and are well known as one of the major groups of antioxidants polyphenols. These compounds are found in various foods and beverages including coffee, tea, wine, grapes, blueberries, pomegranate, and strawberries [17]. They are abundantly distributed in leaves, wood, tree bark, fruit, and roots. Indeed, tannin accounts for 5–10% of the dry weight of plant leaves (**Table 2**) [18].

Tannins have been classified into three major groups: hydrolysable tannin (HT), phlorotannins (PT), and condensed tannin (CT). HTs are compounds with polyol (D-glucose) esterified by phenolic groups and include gallic acid and ellagic acid [19]. CTs are oligomers or polymers of polyhydroxy flavan-3-ol unit (polyphenolic bioflavonoids) and include catechin and epicatechin. HTs are usually distributed in low amounts in plants, while CTs are abundantly or widely distributed in plants (**Table 2**) [20].

Tannins have a wide range of biological and pharmacological activities including antioxidative, anticarcinogenic, anti-inflammatory, antibacterial, cardioprotective and anti-mutagenic activities [17]. Tannin also decreases the blood glucose level in diabetic rats and inhibits adipogenesis in adipose cells [21, 22]. These therapeutic effects are thought to be attributed to the ability of tannins to act as free radical scavengers and to activate antioxidant enzymes, although further studies are needed to confirm this [17]. Because of the versatility of tannins, novel functions of tannins in various chronic diseases have received a great deal of attention because they have great economy and potential ability as therapeutic drugs.

Category	Hydrolyzable tannins	Phlorotannins	Condensed tannins
Structure of basic unit	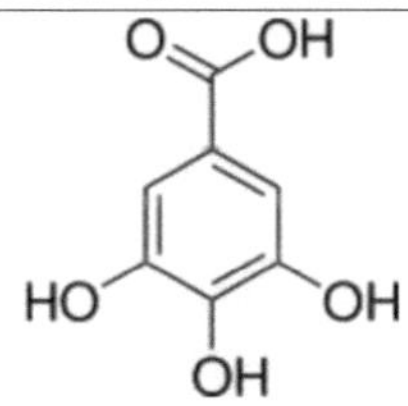	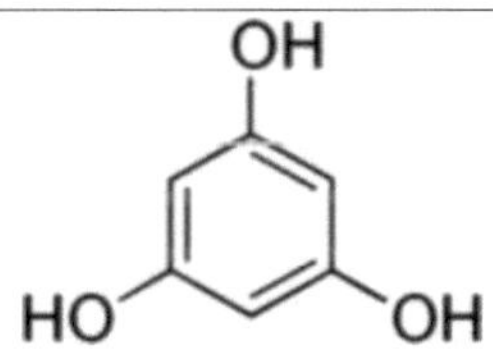	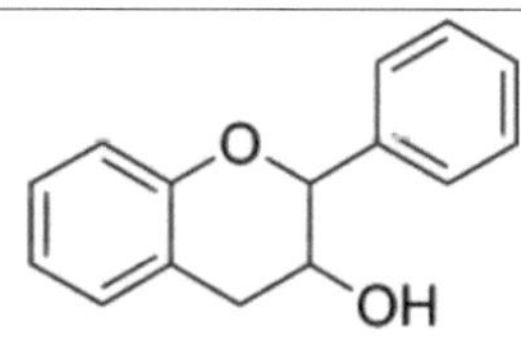
Name of basic unit	Gallic acid	Phloroglucinol	Flavan-3-ol's scaffold
Sources	Pomegranate, strawberries, raspberries, clove, barley, oat, rye, etc.	Brown algae	Coffee, tea, wine, grapes, cranberries, apples, rosemary, etc.
Major compounds	Gallotannins, ellagitannins, punicalagin, ellagic acid, hexahydroxydiphenic acid	Diphlorethol, trifuhalol A, difucophlorethol A, dieckol	Catechin, epicatechin, gallocatechin, epigallocatechin, luteolin, quercetin, arbutin, vanillic acid

Table 2.
Three classifications of tannin [23].

2.2 Laxative effects of natural products containing tannin

2.2.1 Laxative effect of Mareya micrantha Mull. Arg

M. micrantha is a shrub tree that grows in west and central regions of Africa. The leaves of this plant have been used traditionally to treat several diseases including tapeworm infections, gonorrhea, leprosy, and constipation [24, 25]. However, scientific evidence for the therapeutic effects of this plant in several chronic diseases has also been reported. The aqueous extracts of *M. micrantha's* leaf inhibited cardiac contractibility in the hearts of frogs and rats [26, 27], but induced contraction of longitudinal muscle in the guinea pig [28]. The methanol, aqueous, and ethanol extracts of leaves also showed anti-bacterial effects against some pathogens and antiplasmodial activity against *Plasmodium falciparum* [25, 29]. Also, these aqueous leaf extracts of *M. micrantha* had 566.66 kg/body weight of LD_{50} and were classified as low toxic substance [30]. Meanwhile, the aqueous leaf extract of *M. micrantha* contained various phytochemicals including alkaloids, tannins, flavonoids, polyphenols, sterols and polyterpenes although their concentrations were low [31].

Furthermore, the aqueous leaf extract of *M. micrantha* enhanced the gastrointestinal motility, intestinal water secretion, intestinal ion secretion, and stool output in a dose-dependent manner (100, 200 and 400 mg/kg) in Wistar rats. Similar effects were observed in The loperamode (Lop)-induced constipation model. The total stool number and weight were significantly increased after treatment with the aqueous leaf extract of *M. micrantha* (**Table 3**). The laxative effects of this product at 400 mg/kg were very similar to those of 5 mg/kg of sodium picosulfate [31].

2.2.2 Laxative effects of A. ferox Mill

A. ferox is an arborescent perennial shrub that is widely distributed in Southern Cape, Eastern Cape, Southern parts of KwaZulu Natal, the Free State and Lesotho [10]. This plant has been widely used in traditional medicine because of its healing properties against several human diseases [32], particularly tooth abscesses [33], sexually transmitted infections [34], wound healing [35], arthritis and rheumatism [36], conjunctivitis and eye ailments [37] and as an insect repellant [38].

The acetone extract of the whole leaf of *A. ferox Mill*. contained phenols (70.33%), flavonols (35.2%), proanthocyanidins (171.06%) and alkaloids (60.9%), while the ethanol extract contained the same compounds at values of 70.24%, 12.53%, 76.7% and 23.76%, respectively. Their concentrations in aqueous extract were lower than those in acetone and ethanol. In contrast, tannin levels were consistently 0.014–0.027% in all the solvent extracts [39].

Treatment	Dose	Weight of feces (g)
Control	5 mL/kg	0.938 ± 0.45
Sodium picosulfate	5 mg/kg	3.84 ± 0.62**
MAR	100 mg/kg	2.602 ± 0.33
MAR	200 mg/kg	2.806 ± 0.42*
MAR	400 mg/kg	3.507 ± 0.45**

Values are expressed as mean ± S.E.M (n = 5).
**p < 0.05 compared to control group.*
***p < 0.01 compared to control group.*

Table 3.
Laxative effect of M. micrantha aqueous extract (MAR) on Lop-induced constipation model [30].

Although various effects of this plant have been reported previously, scientific evidence for laxative effects of *Aloe ferox* was reported recently. The aqueous extract of *A. ferox* remarkably enhanced the water intake and the number, water content and weight of stools in the Lop-induced constipation model (**Table 4**). Also, a significant increase in the gastrointestinal transit ratio was induced by the administration of aqueous extract of *A. ferox*. These effects of this plant at 200 mg/kg were comparable to those of senokot [10]. Moreover, this extract was not induced any significant toxic effect on the hematological parameters for kidney and the liver function at 50, 100 and 200 mg/kg body weight for 7 days [40].

2.3 Laxative effects of *Urginea indica* Kunth

U. indica belongs to family Liliaceae and is distributed in western Himalayas and Coromandel Coast [41]. This plant was traditionally used to treat skin diseases, asthma, cough, bronchitis, calculous affections, rheumatism, leprosy, paralytic affection, internal pain, and scabies [42–44]. The bulbs of this plant were applied to relieve constipation and indigestion, to prevent burning sensations, and to remove corns and warts [41, 44, 45]. Also, its antifungal, antiangiogenic and pro-apoptotic effects were reported previously [46, 47]. Various phytochemical components including alkaloids, tannins and coumarins were detected in the crude aqueous-methanol extract of *U. indica* [48].

Laxative effects of *U. indica* have been examined in rabbits, guinea pigs and mice. The charcoal meal transit was accelerated in the small intestine of mice treated with *U. indica*. The total number of stools also increased in a dose-dependent manner in *U. indica*-treated mice. Furthermore, concentration-dependent spasmogenic effects of crude extract of *U. indica* were detected in guinea-pig ileum and rabbit jejunum (**Figure 1**) [48]. Moreover, this study provided the first evidence that the stimulant effect of *U. indica* was mediated by the activation of muscarinic receptors initiating the prokinetic effect [48].

Parameters	Normal control	Constipated control	Constipated + *A. ferox* (mg/kg body weight)			Senokot
			50	100	200	
Feed intake	17.18 ± 1.36^a	19.23 ± 3.86^a	19.90 ± 1.61^a	20.54 ± 1.38^a	17.80 ± 1.60^a	19.97 ± 3.31^a
Water intake	19.62 ± 2.22^a	11.72 ± 2.47^b	16.57 ± 2.05^a	17.24 ± 0.17^a	19.79 ± 2.33^a	18.14 ± 0.61^a
Number of fecal pellet	73.57 ± 4.39^a	38.20 ± 2.21^b	45.43 ± 1.90^c	57.57 ± 1.62^d	69.83 ± 4.49^a	63.00 ± 3.11^a
Water content of fecal pellet (ml)	14.40 ± 0.08^a	1.04 ± 0.09^b	1.75 ± 0.21^c	1.95 ± 0.11^c	2.25 ± 0.21^d	2.09 ± 0.06^d
Weight of fecal pellet (g)	7.14 ± 0.23^a	3.34 ± 0.38^b	5.72 ± 0.18^c	7.42 ± 0.33^a	8.10 ± 0.72^a	7.31 ± 0.25^a
Body weight gain (g)	15.30 ± 1.00^a	33.80 ± 1.00^b	14.20 ± 0.71^a	13.20 ± 2.16^a	12.50 ± 1.85^a	15.35 ± 1.21^a

Data are mean ± SD values (n = 4). Row values with different superscripts than the control are significantly different (P < 0.05).

Table 4.
Laxative effect of aqueous extract of A. ferox in constipated rats [31].

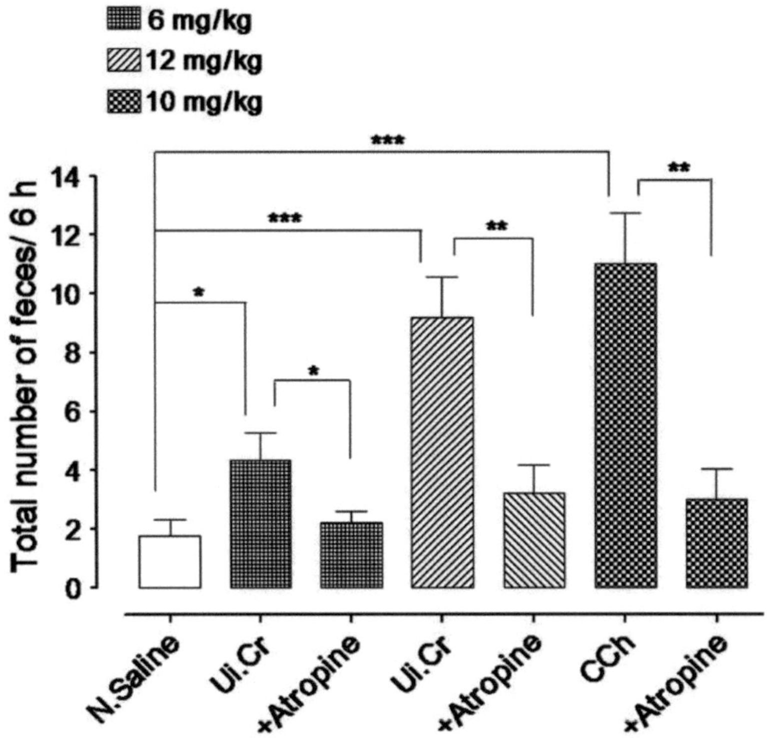

Figure 1.
*Effect of U. indica crude extract (Ui.Cr) and carbachol (CCh) on fecal number in the presence and absence of atropine. Values are expressed as mean ± SEM, n = 6. *p < 0.05 compared to control, **p < 0.01 compared to control and ***p < 0.001 compared to control [47]. Abbreviations: N. Saline, normal saline; +atropine, atropine cotreatment.*

2.4 Laxative effects of *Fumaria parviflora*

F. parviflora is an annual flowering plant and is widely distributed in many parts of the world including the Middle East and South Asia [43, 49]. The aqueous-methanol extract of this plant contained alkaloids such as adlumidiceine, coptisine, fumariline, parfumine, protopine [50], fumaranine, fumaritine, paprafumicin, paprarine [51], fumarophycine, cryptopine, sanactine, stylopine, bicuculline, adlumine, perfumidine and dihydrosanguirine [52]. Also, the aqueous-methanol extract of *F. parviflora* contained alkaloid, saponins, anthraquinones and tannins [53].

In Greco-Arab traditional medicine, this plant was used to treat indigestion, constipation, abdominal cramps and diarrhea [43, 49]. Recently, the laxative and prokinetic activity of this plant were investigated in three different animals. The charcoal meal GI transit, defecation and number of wet stools were enhanced in a dose-dependent manner in mice. Also, this plant induced a concentration-dependent, atropine-sensitive stimulatory effect both in mouse tissues (jejunum and ileum) and rabbit jejunum (**Figure 2**) [14].

2.5 Laxative effects of *Phyllanthus emblica*

P. emblica is a natural plant distributed in most areas of the Sind and Punjab provinces of Pakistan [43]. Most parts of this plant including the fruit, seed, leaves, root, bark and flowers are used in the herbal preparations due to their high phenolic contents [54].

The leaves of *P. emblica* contain tannins like glucogallin, corilagin, chebulagic acid, tannins emblicanins A and B [55], and apigenin glucoside [56]. The roots of this plant

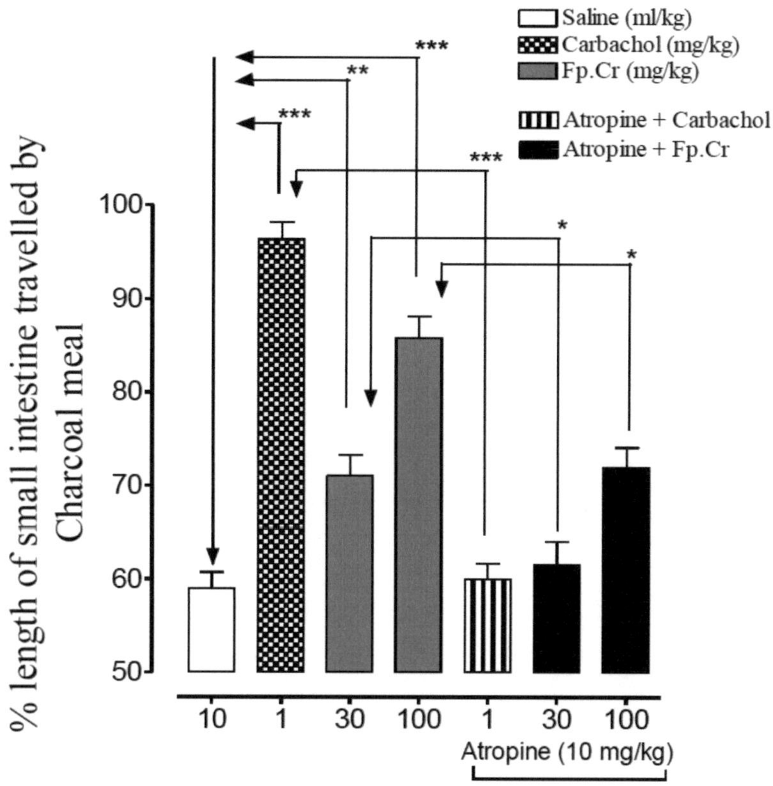

Figure 2.
Laxative effects of F. parviflora (Fp.Cr) crude extract on travel of charcoal meal through small intestine of mice, in the absence and presence of atropine. $^{*}p < 0.05$ *compared with control,* $^{**}p < 0.01$ *compared to control and* $^{***}p < 0.001$ *compared to control [52].*

contain norsesquiterpenoid glycosides (4′-hydroxyphyllaemblicin B, phyllaemblicins E and F, phyllaemblic acid, phyllaemblicin A, B and C) [57], quercetin and b-sitosterol [58]. The leaves are known to have multiple health benefits including gastroprotective, anti-ulcerogenic, hypolipidemic and antidiabetic [59], antioxidant [60], hepatoprotective [61], antihypertensive [62], anti-inflammatory [63], antidiarrheal and antispasmodic [64] activities. But, the crude extract of dried fruits showed laxative effects that increased charcoal meal GI transit, the mean weight of defecation, and the number of stools. The crude extracts and aqueous fraction induced dose-dependent and partially atropine-sensitive contraction in isolated guinea-pig ileum and rabbit jejunum, while the petroleum fraction showed full atropine-sensitive contraction. In contrast, spasmolytic activity was detected in the ethylacetate and chloroform fractions of this plant (**Figure 3**) [54]. Furthermore, extracts from the leaves of *P. emblica* showed 9.911 g/kg of LD50 and the indexes of thymus and spleen in the *P. emblica* extract–treated groups had no markedly difference [65].

2.6 Laxative effects of Galla Rhois

The laxative effect of Galla Rhois as a natural product containing high concentrations of tannin was investigated by Kim et al. [66]. Galla Rhois is an excrescence formed by parasitic aphids, primarily *Schlechtendalia chinensis Bell*, on the leaf of sumac, *Rhus javanica* (Anacardiaceae) (**Figure 4**) [67]. This product has been widely used for treatment of various diseases including diarrhea, seminal emissions, excessive sweating, boil, some skin diseases, bleeding, and chronic cough because of its

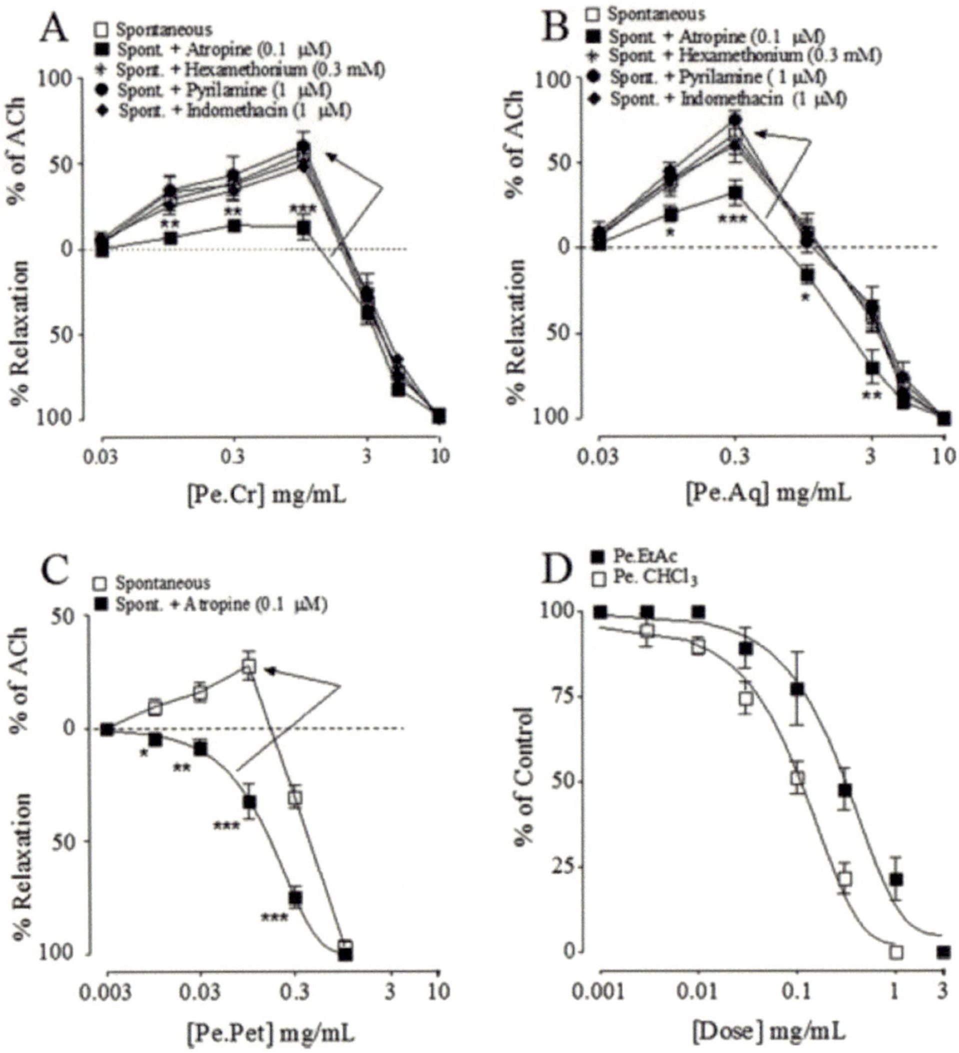

Figure 3.
*Stimulant and relaxant effects of several extracts and fractions of P. emblica. The concentration of acetylcholine (Ach) was measured in rabbit jejunum after treatment with (A) the crude extract (Pe.Cr), (B) the aqueous extract (Pe.Aq) in the absence and presence of atropine, hexamethonium, pyrilamine and indomethacin, (C) the effect of petroleum fraction (Pe.Pet) in the absence and presence of atropine, (D) the ethyl acetate (Pe.EtAc) and chloroform (Pe.CHCl$_3$) fractions. Values shown represent mean ± SEM of 6–7 determinations. *p < 0.05 compared with control, **p < 0.01 compared with control, and ***p < 0.001 compared with control [54]. Abbreviations: Spont., spontaneous.*

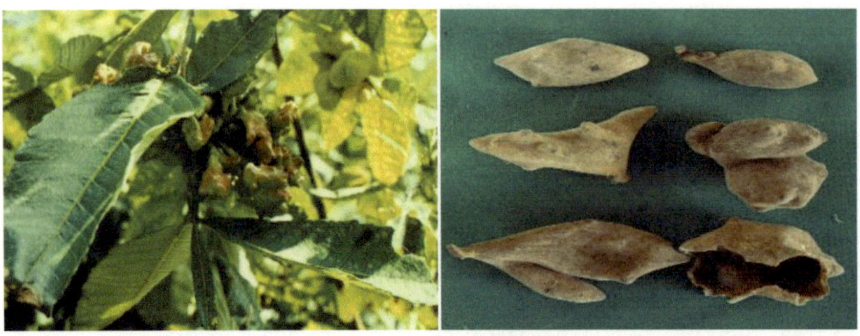

Figure 4.
Living and dry forms of Galla Rhois [76].

ethnopharmacological properties [67–69]. In particular, the antibacterial effects of Galla Rhois have been detected against many pathogenic bacteria such as *Salmonella* spp., *Escherichia coli* and *Eimeria tenella* [70–72], while anti-inflammatory activity is observed in lipopolysaccharide (LPS)-stimulated RAW264.7 macrophages [73]. Also, Galla Rhois shows anticancer activity against nasopharyngeal carcinoma cells [74] and improves sensorimotor function in a cerebral ischemia rat model [75].

Meanwhile, the ingredients in gallotannin-enriched Galla Rhois (GEGR) have been measured by UV-Vis spectra and HPLC analyses. They consist of gallotannin (69.2%), gallic acid (26.6%) and methyl gallate (4.2%) (**Figure 5**) [66].

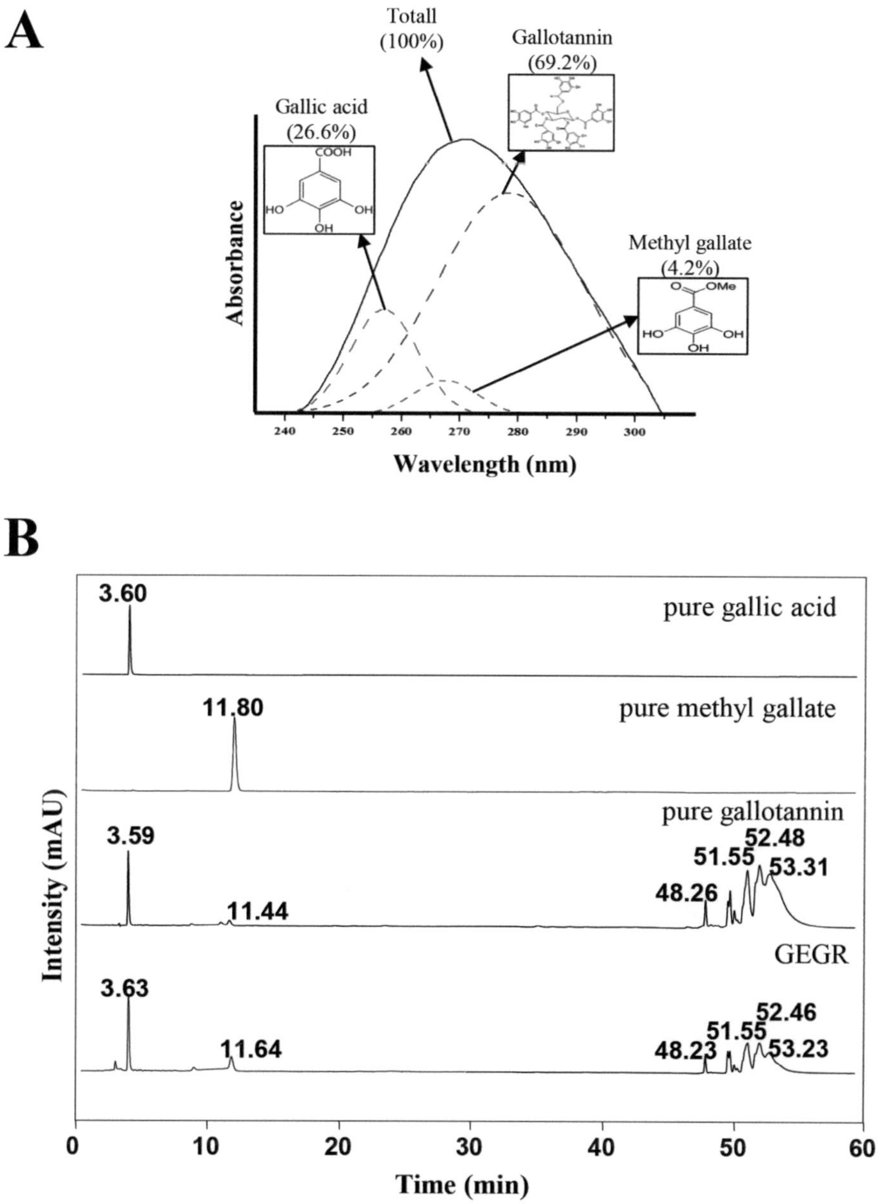

Figure 5.
Ingredients of GEGR. Concentration of major components. (A) The levels of gallotannin, gallic acid and methyl gallate in GEGR were analyzed based on their UV-vis spectra. (B) HPLC chromatograms of pure gallic acid (commercial chemical), pure methyl gallate (commercial chemical), pure gallotannin (commercial chemical), and GEGR extract [66].

In the Lop-induced constipation model, the number and weight of stools was almost recovered in the GEGR-treated groups compared to those in the untreated and vehicle-treated groups. Also, significant alterations in the thickness of the

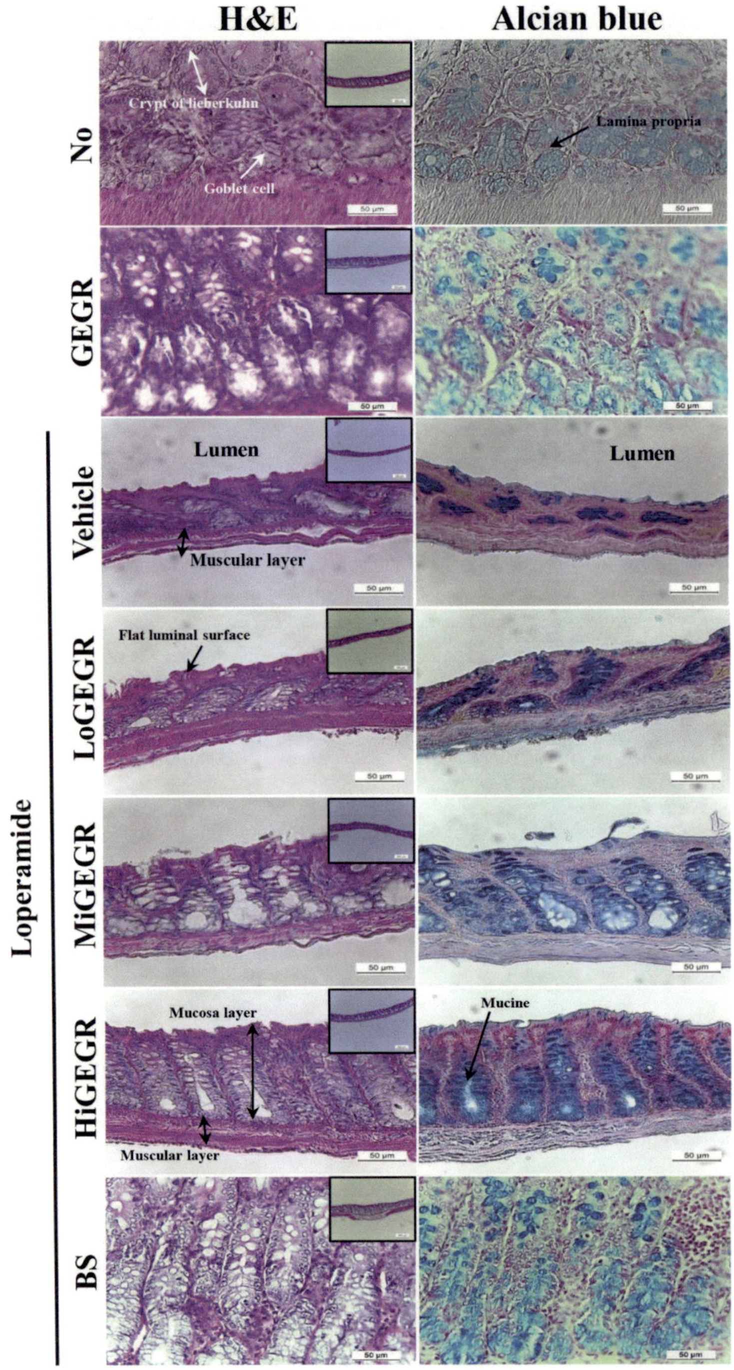

Figure 6.
Recovery effects of GEGR on the histological structure of transverse colon. After collecting the transverse colon from the subset group, these tissues were stained with H&E solution and Alcian blue. Their morphological features were observed at 100X (upper corner in left column) and 200x (left column and right column) using a light microscope [66]. Abbreviations: No, no treated group; BS, bisacodyl-treated group; LoGEGR, low level of GEGR-treated group; MiGEGR, medium level of GEGR-treated group; HiGEGR, high level of GEGR-treated group.

mucosa, muscle, and flat luminal surface, as well as in the ability to secrete mucin, were detected in the transverse colon of constipated SD rats (**Figure 6**) [66].

Furthermore, the mechanism of GEGR action during the laxative effects was investigated on the downstream signaling pathway of the muscarinic acetylcholine receptor. The Lop + GEGR-treated group was remarkably recovered compared to the Lop + vehicle-treated group. A similar pattern was detected for the phosphorylation levels of protein kinase C (PKC) and phosphoinositide 3-kinase (PI3K), the levels of Gα expression and the inositol triphosphate (IP3) concentration after GEGR treatment (**Figure 7**) [66]. However, GEGR did not induce any significant toxic effect on liver and kidney organs of ICR at doses of 1000 mg/kg body weight/day [69].

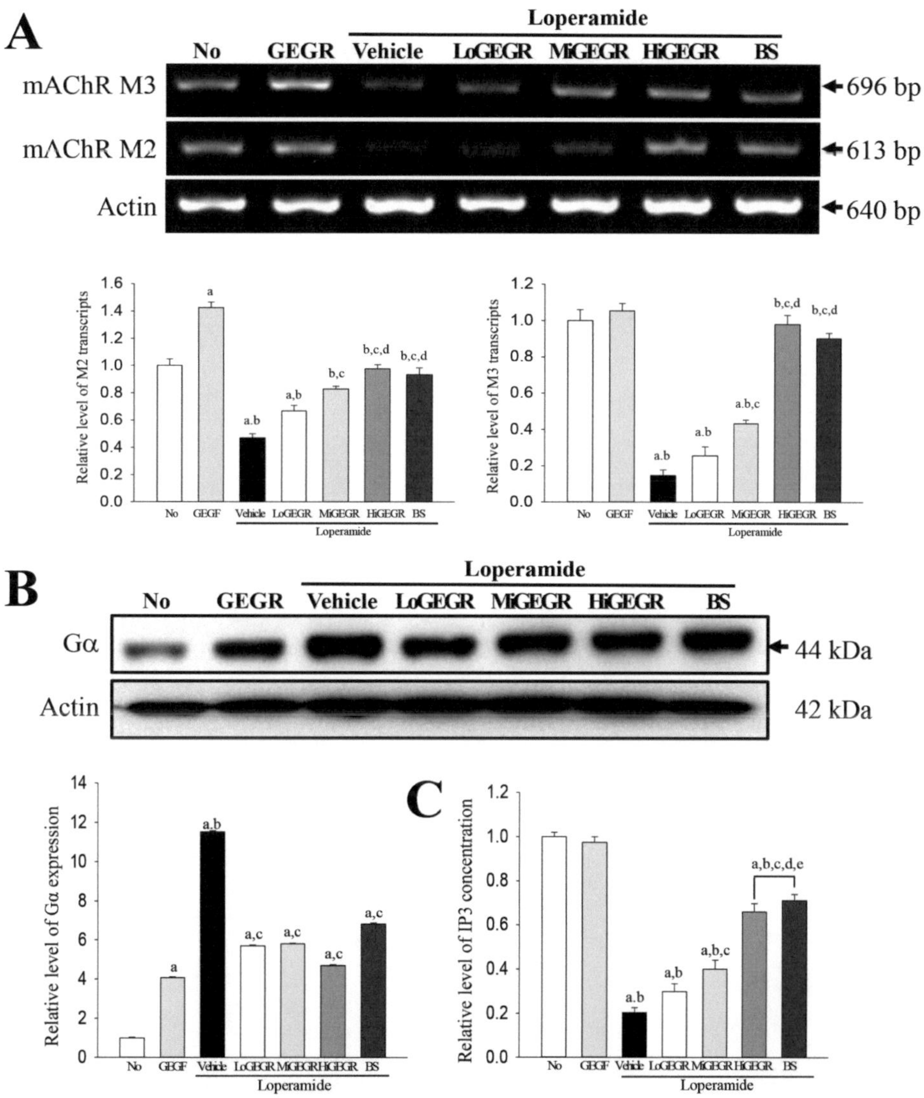

Figure 7.
Recovery effects of GEGR and mAChRs transcript and their downstream effectors. (A) The levels of mAChR M2 and M3 transcripts were measured by RT-PCR using specific primers. (B) The expression of Gα was measured by Western blotting using HRP-labeled anti-rabbit IgG antibody. (C) The IP3 concentration in total tissue homogenates was quantified by enzyme-linked immunosorbent assay. The relative levels of protein and transcript of mAChRs were calculated based on the intensity of actin protein and mRNA [66]. Abbreviations: No, no treated group; BS, bisacodyl-treated group; LoGEGR, low level of GEGR-treated group; MiGEGR, medium level of GEGR-treated group; HiGEGR, high level of GEGR-treated group; mAChR, muscarinic acetylcholine receptor.

3. Conclusions

Various bioactive molecules with therapeutic effects on human diseases have been isolated from many traditional plants including medicinal plants, aromatic plants, vegetables, and fruits [77]. Among these, tannins are some of the many

Name of natural products	Constituents	Laxative effects	Reference
M. micrantha (Benth.) Mull. Arg.	Alkaloids, tannins, flavonoid, polyphenols, sterols and polyterpenes	- Increase the gastrointestinal motility - Increase the intestinal water secretion - Increase the intestinal ion secretion - Increase the stools parameters	[31]
A. ferox Mill.	Phenols, flavonoid, proanthocyanidins, alkaloids and tannins	- Increase the stools parameters - Increase the gastrointestinal transit ratio	[10]
U. indica Kunth.	Alkaloids, tannins and coumarins	- Increase the gastrointestinal transit ratio - Increase the stools parameters - Show the concentration-dependent spasmogenic effects	[48]
F. parviflora	Alkaloids, saponins, anthraquinones and tannins	- Increase the gastrointestinal transit ratio - Increase the stools parameters - Show the concentration-dependent spasmogenic effects	[52]
S. macranthera	Flavonoids, tannins and coumarins	- Increase the gastrointestinal motility - Increase the stools parameters	[15]
P. emblica	Alkaloids, saponins, tannins, terpenes, flavonoid, sterol and coumarins	- Increase the gastrointestinal transit ratio - Increase the stools parameters - Show the concentration-dependent spasmogenic effects	[54]
Galla Rhois	Gallic acid, methyl gallate and gallotannin	- Increase the stools parameters - Recovery the histopathological structure - Increase the mucin secretion ability - Recovery the mAChRs downstream signaling pathway	[66]

Table 5.
Summary of natural products containing tannin and their laxative effects.

phytochemicals and have various pharmacological activities against many chronic diseases such as cardiovascular disease, inflammatory diseases, cancer, obesity and diabetes due to their high antioxidant activity [17]. Tannins have also received a great deal of attention as novel therapeutic drugs for use in the treatment of chronic constipation and its related conditions. In an effort to identify candidate drugs for the treatment of chronic constipation and verify the role of tannins as key laxatives, this review describes some of the evidence supporting the use of natural products containing tannin as laxatives in several constipation models. Excellent laxative effects were detected for extracts of *M. micrantha*, *A. ferox*, *U. indica*, *F. parviflora*, *S. macranthera* and *P. emblica*. In particular, Galla Rhois, which contains a high concentration of gallotannin (69.2%), remarkably improved the symptoms of constipation (**Table 5**).

In conclusion, this review provides evidence correlating the laxative effects with natural products containing tannin, although the mechanism of action has not been completely verified. Therefore, tannins may be a viable laxative treatment of humans. However, more research is needed to verify the molecular mechanism and long-term effects of each tannin type.

Acknowledgements

I would like to express my gratitude to my students, including JE Kim, ML Lee, JJ Park, BR Song, HR Kim, JW Park, MJ Kang, HJ Choi and SJ Bae, for helping to compile this paper and for helping with the graphics and charts herein. This review was supported by the Basic Science Research Program through the National Research Foundation of Korea (NRF) funded by the Ministry of Education (2017R1D1A3B03032631).

Author details

Dae Youn Hwang
Department of Biomaterials Science, College of Natural Resources and Life Science, Pusan National University, Miryang, Korea

*Address all correspondence to: dyhwang@pusan.ac.kr

References

[1] El-Salhy M, Svensen R, Hatlebakk JG, Gilja OH, Hausken T. Chronic constipation and treatment options (review). Molecular Medicine Reports. 2014;**9**(1):3-8

[2] Walia R, Mahajan L, Steffen R. Recent advances in chronic constipation. Current Opinion in Pediatrics. 2009;**21**:661-666. DOI: 10.1097/MOP.0b013e32832ff241

[3] Emmanuel AV, Tack J, Quigley EM, Talley NJ. Pharmacological management of constipation. Neurogastroenterology and Motility. 2009;**21**:41-54. DOI: 10.1111/j.1365-2982.2009.01403.x

[4] Leung FW. Etiologic factors of chronic constipation: Review of the scientific evidence. Digestive Diseases and Sciences. 2007;**52**:313-316. DOI: 10.1007/s10620-006-9298-7

[5] Liu LWC. Chronic constipation: Current treatment options. Canadian Journal of Gastroenterology. 2011;**25**(suppl B):22B-28B

[6] Hussain ZH, Everhart K, Lacy BE. Treatment of chronic constipation: Prescription medications and surgical therapies. Gastroenterology & Hepatology. 2015;**11**(2):104-114

[7] Tzavella K, Riepl RL, Klauser AG, Voderholzer WA, Schindbeck NE, Müller-Lissner SA. Decreased substance P levels in rectal biopsies from patients with slow transit constipation. European Journal of Gastroenterology & Hepatology. 1996;**8**:1207-1211

[8] Schiller LR. The therapy of constipation. Alimentary Pharmacology & Therapeutics. 2001;**15**:749-763. DOI: 10.1046/j.1365-2036.2001.00982.x

[9] Quigley EM, Vandeplassche L, Kerstens R, Ausma J. Clinical trial: The efficacy, impact on quality of life, and safety and tolerability of prucalopride in severe chronic constipation—A 12-week, randomized, double-blind, placebo-controlled study. Alimentary Pharmacology & Therapeutics. 2009;**29**:315-328. DOI: 10.1111/j.1365-2036.2008.03884.x

[10] Wintola OA, Sunmonu TO, Afolayan AJ. The effect of *Aloe ferox* Mill. in the treatment of loperamide-induced constipation in Wistar rats. BMC Gastroenterology. 2010;**10**:95-99. DOI: 10.1186/1471-230X-10-95

[11] Kakino M, Izuta H, Ito T, Tsuruma K, Araki Y, Shimazawa M, et al. Agarwood induced laxative effects via acetylcholine receptors on loperamide-induced constipation in mice. Bioscience, Biotechnology, and Biochemistry. 2010;**74**:1550-1555. DOI: 10.1271/bbb.100122

[12] Lee HY, Kim JH, Jeung HW, Lee CU, Kim DS, Li B, et al. Effects of *Ficus carica* paste on loperamide-induced constipation in rats. Food and Chemical Toxicology. 2012;**50**:895-902. DOI: 10.1016/j.fct.2011.12.001

[13] Han SH, Park K, Kim EY, Ahn SH, Lee HS, Suh HJ. Cactus (*Opuntia humifusa*) water extract ameliorates loperamide-induced constipation in rats. BMC Complementary and Alternative Medicine. 2017;**17**(1): 49-56. DOI: 10.1186/s12906-016-1552-8

[14] Méité S, Bahi C, Yéo D, Datté JY, Djaman JA, N'guessan DJ. Laxative activities of *Mareya micrantha* (Benth.) Müll. Arg. (Euphorbiaceae) leaf aqueous extract in rats. BMC Complementary and Alternative Medicine. 2010;**10**:7. DOI: 10.1186/1472-6882-10-7

[15] Guarize L, Costa JC, Dutra LB, Mendes RF, Lima IVA, Scio E. Anti-inflammatory, laxative and

intestinal motility effects of *Senna macranthera* leaves. Natural Product Research. 2012;**26**:331-343. DOI: 10.1080/14786411003754264

[16] Kim JE, Lee YJ, Kwak MH, Ko J, Hong JT, Hwang DY. Aqueous extracts of *Liriope platyphylla* induced significant laxative effects on loperamide-induced constipation of SD rats. BMC Complementary and Alternative Medicine. 2013;**13**:333-344. DOI: 10.1186/1472-6882-13-333

[17] Kumari M, Jain S. Tannins: An antinutrient with positive effect to manage diabetes. Research Journal of Recent Sciences. 2012;**1**(12):1-8

[18] Barbehenn RV, Peter Constabel C. Tannins in plant-herbivore interactions. Phytochemistry. 2011;**72**(13):1551-1565. DOI: 10.1016/j.phytochem.2011.01.040

[19] Hemingway RW, Karchesy JJ. Chemistry and Significance of Condensed Tannins. Vol. 113. London: Pleum Press; 2014

[20] Koleckar V, Kubikova K, Rehakova Z, Kuca K, Jun D, Jahodar L, et al. Condensed and hydrolysable tannins as antioxidants influencing the health. Mini Reviews in Medicinal Chemistry. 2008;**8**(5):436-447. DOI: 10.2174/138955708784223486

[21] Pinent M, Blay M, Blade MC, Salvado MJ, Arola L, Ardevol A. Grape seed-derived procyanidins have an antihyperglycemic effect in streptozotocin-induced diabetic rats and insulinomimetic activity in insulin-sensitive cell lines. Endocrinology. 2004;**145**:4985-4990. DOI: 10.1210/en.2004-0764

[22] Muthusamy VS, Anand S, Sangeetha KN, Sujatha S, Lakshmi BABS. Tannins present in *Cichorium intybus* enhance glucose uptake and inhibit adipogenesis in 3T3-L1 adipocytes through PTP1B inhibition. Chemico-Biological Interactions. 2008;**174**:69-78. DOI: 10.1016/j.cbi.2008.04.016

[23] Kirkea DA, Smyth TJ, Rai DK, Kenny O, Stengel DB. The chemical and antioxidant stability of isolated low molecular weight phlorotannins. Food Chemistry. 2011;**15**:1104-1112. DOI: 10.1016/j.foodchem.2016.11.050

[24] N'guessan K. Thèse de Doctorat 3ème cycle. Université d'Abidjan-Cocody, Botanique et biologie. Contribution à l'étude ethnobotanique chez les Krobou de la souspréfecture d'Agboville (Côte d'Ivoire). 1995

[25] Mac Foy CA, Cline EI. *In vitro* antibacterial activities of three plants used in traditional medicine in Sierra Leone. Journal of Ethnopharmacology. 1990;**28**:323-327, 90083-90086. DOI: 10.1016/0378-8741(90)

[26] Guede-guina F, Tsai CS, Smith MO, Vangah MM, Washington B, Ochillo RF. The use of isolated functional heart to pharmacologically characterize active ingredient in the aqueous extracts of *Mareya micrantha*. Journal of Ethnopharmacology. 1995;**45**:19-26. DOI: 10.1016/0378-8741(94)01190-B

[27] Abo KJ-C, Aka KJ, Ehile EE, Guede Guina F, Traore F. Effets cholinergiques d'un extrait aqueux brut de Mareya micrantha (Euphorbiacée) sur la pression et d'activité cardiaque. La Revue de Médecine et de Pharmacie. 2000;**5**:11-20

[28] Tsai CS, Guede Guina F, Smith MO, Vangah MM, Ochillo RF. Isolation of cholinergic active ingredients in aqueous extracts of *Mareya micrantha* using the longitudinal muscle of isolated Guinea-pig ileum as a pharmacological activity marker. Journal of Ethnopharmacology. 1995;**45**:215-222. DOI: 10.1016/0378-8741(94)01219-P

[29] Zirihi GN, Mambu L, Guédé-Guina F, Bodo B, Grellier P. *In vitro*

antiplasmodial activity and cytotoxicity of 33 West African plants used for the treatment of malaria. Journal of Ethnopharmacology. 2005;**98**:281-285. DOI: 10.1016/j.jep.2005.01.004

[30] Dosso M, Meite S, Yeo D, Traore F, Diaman AJ, N'guessan JD. Cholinergic and histaminergic activites of the aqueous extract of mareya micrantha (Benth) *Mareya micrantha* (Benth). Müll Arg (Euphorbiaceae). Asian Journal of Chemistry. 2013;**8**(1):24-32. DOI: 10.3923/ajb.2013.24.32

[31] Méité S, Bahi C, Yéo D, Datté JY, Djaman JA, N'guessan DJ. Laxative activities of *Mareya micrantha* (Benth.). Müll. Arg. (Euphorbiaceae) leaf aqueous extract in rats. BMC Complementary and Alternative Medicine. 2010;**10**. DOI: 7. DOI:10.1186/1472-6882-10-7

[32] Zahn M, Trinh T, Jeong ML, Wang D, Abeysingbe P, Jia Q. A revised-phase high performance liquid chromatographic method for the determination of aloesin A and anthraquinone of *Aloc ferox*. Phytochemical Analysis. 2007;**19**:122-126. DOI: 10.1002/pca.1024

[33] Githens TS. Drug Plants of Africa. Philadelphia: University of Pennsylvania Press; 1979. 50 p

[34] Kambizi L, Goosen BM, Taylor MB, Afolayan AJ. Anti-viral effects of aqueous extracts of *Aloe ferox* and *Withania somnifera* on herpes simplex virus type 1 in cell culture. South African Journal of Science. 2007;**103**:359-360

[35] Grierson DS, Afolayan AJ. An ethnobotanical study of plants used for the treatment of wounds in the Eastern Cape, South Africa. Journal of Ethnopharmacology. 1999;**67**:327-332. DOI: 10.1016/S0378-8741(99)00082-3

[36] Van Wyk B-E, Van Oudtshoorn B, Gericke N. Medicinal Plants of South Africa Pretoria. 2nd ed. South Africa: Briza Publication; 1997. 42 p

[37] Crouch NR, Symmonds R, Spring A, Diederichs N. Fact sheet for growing popular medicinal plant species. In: Commercializing Medicinal plants: A Southern African Guide. Stellenbosch: Sun Press; 2006. pp. 100-102

[38] Watt J, Breyer-Brandwijk MG. Medicinal and Poisonous Plants of Southern and Eastern Africa. 2nd ed. London: Livingstone; 1962

[39] Wintola OA, Afolayan AJ. Phytochemical constituents and antioxidant activities of the whole leaf extract of *Aloe ferox* Mill. Pharmacognosy Magazine. 2011;**7**(28):325-333. DOI: 10.4103/0973-1296.90414

[40] Wintola OA, Sunmonu T, Afolayan AJ. Toxicological evaluation of aqueous extract of *Aloe foerox* Mill. In loperamide-induced constipated rats. Human & Experimental Toxicology. 2011;**30**(5):425-431. DOI: 10.1177/0960327110372647

[41] Kapoor LD. Handbook of Ayurvedic Medicinal Plants: Herbal Reference Library. Australia: CRC Press Boca Raton; 1990. pp. 324-328

[42] Kirtikar KR, Basu BD. Indian Medicinal Plants. India: Periodical Experts Book Agency; 1988. 2331 p

[43] Baquar SR. Medicinal and Poisonous Plants of Pakistan. 2nd ed. Printas: Karachi; 1989. p. 61. 209-210

[44] Prajapati ND, Purohit SS, Sharma AK, Kumar T. A Hand Book of Medicinal Plants—A Complete Source Book. New Delhi: Agrobios; 2003. 32 p

[45] Usmanghani K, Saeed A, Alam MT. Indusyunic Medicine. Karachi: University of Karachi Press; 1997.

[46] Shenoy SR, Kameshwari MN, Swaminathan S, Gupta MN. Major antifungal activity from the bulbs of indian squill *Urginea indica* is a chitinase. Biotechnology Progress. 2006;**22**: 631-637. DOI: 10.1021/bp050305n

[47] Deepak AV, Salimath BP. Antiangiogenic and proapoptotic activity of a novel glycoprotein from *Urginea indica* is mediated by NF-kappaB and Caspase activated DNase in ascites tumor model. Biochimie. 2006;**88**:297-307. DOI: 10.1007/s11010-005-7717-2

[48] Abbas S, Bashir S, Khan A, Mehmood MH, Gilani AH. Gastrointestinal stimulant effect of *Urginea indica* Kunth. and involvement of muscarinic receptors. Phytotherapy Research. 2012;**26**(5):704-708. DOI: 10.1002/ptr.3634

[49] Mossa JS, Al-Yahya MA, AlMeshal IA. Medicinal Plants of Saudi Arabia. Riyadh: King Saud University Libraries Publications; 1987

[50] Popova ME, Simanek V, Dolejs L, Smysl B, Preininger V. Alkaloids from *Fumaria parviflora* and *Fumaria kralikii*. Planta Medica. 1982;**45**:120-122. DOI: 10.1055/s-2007-971259

[51] Rahman AU, Khati MK, Choudhary MI, Sener B. Chemical constituents of *Fumaria indica*. Fitoterapia. 1992;**63**:129-135

[52] Rehman N, Mehmood MH, Al-Rehaily AJ, Mothana RAA, Gilani AH: Species and tissue-specificity of prokinetic, laxative and spasmodic effects of *Fumaria parviflora*. BMC Complementary and Alternative Medicine. 2012;**12**:16. DOI: 10.1186/1472-6882-12-16

[53] Suau R, Cabezudo B, Rico R, Najera F, Lopez-Romero JM. Direct determination of alkaloid contents in Fumaria species by GC-MS. Phytochemical Analysis. 2002;**13**:363-367. DOI: 10.1002/pca.669

[54] Mehmood MH, Rehman A, Rehman N, Gilani AH. Studies on Prokinetic, laxative and spasmodic activities of *Phyllanthus emblica* in experimental animals. Phytotherapy Research. 2013;**27**:1054-1060. DOI: 10.1002/ptr.4821

[55] Majeed M, Bhat B, Jadhav AN, Srivastava JS, Nagabhushanam K. Ascorbic acid and tannins from *Emblica officinalis* Gaertn. fruits—A revisit. Journal of Agricultural and Food Chemistry. 2009;**57**:220-225. DOI: 10.1021/jf802900b

[56] El-Desouky SK, Ryu SY, Kim YK. A new cytotoxic acylated apigenin glucoside from *Phyllanthus emblica* L. Natural Product Research. 2008;**22**:91-95. DOI: 10.1080/14786410701590236

[57] Liu Q, Wang YF, Chen RJ, Zhang MY, Wang YF, Yang CR, et al. Anti-coxsackie virus B3 norsesquiterpenoids from the roots of *Phyllanthus emblica*. Journal of Natural Products. 2009;**72**:969-972. DOI: 10.1021/np800792d

[58] Thakur RS, Puri HS, Husain A. Major Medicinal Plants of India. India: CIMAP; 1989. Lucknow

[59] Krishnaveni M, Mirunalini S. Therapeutic potential of *Phyllanthus emblica* (amla): The ayurvedic wonder. Journal of Basic and Clinical Physiology and Pharmacology. 2010;**21**:93-105. DOI: 10.1515/JBCPP.2010.21.1.93

[60] Sharma A, Sharma MK, Kumar M. Modulatory role of *Emblica officinalis* fruit extract against arsenic induced oxidative stress in Swiss albino mice. Chemico-Biological Interactions. 2009;**180**:20-30. DOI: 10.1016/j.cbi.2009.01.012

[61] Srirama R, Deepak HB, Senthilkumar U, Ravikanth G, Gurumurthy BR, Shivanna MB, et al. Hepatoprotective activity of *Indian Phyllanthus*. Pharmaceutical Biology. 2012;**50**:948-953. DOI: 10.3109/13880209.2011.649858

[62] Bhatia J, Tabassum F, Sharma AK, Bharti S, Golechha M, Joshi S, et al. *Emblica officinalis* exerts antihypertensive effect in a rat model of DOCA-salt induced hypertension: Role of (p) eNOS, NO and oxidative stress. Cardiovascular Toxicology. 2011;**11**:272-279. DOI: 10.1007/s12012-011-9122-2

[63] Nicolis E, Lampronti I, Dechecchi MC, Borgatti M, Tamanini A, Bianchi N, et al. Pyrogallol, an active compound from the medicinal plant *Emblica officinalis*, regulates expression of pro-inflammatory genes in bronchial epithelial cells. International Immunology. 2008;**8**:1672-1680. DOI: 10.1016/j.intimp.2008.08.001

[64] Mehmood MH, Siddiqi HS, Gilani AH. The antidiarrheal and spasmolytic activities of *Phyllanthus emblica* Linn. Are mediated through dual blockade of muscarinic receptors and calcium channels. Journal of Ethnopharmacology. 2011;**133**: 856-865. DOI: 10.1016/j.jep.2010.11.023

[65] Zhong ZG, Luo XF, Huang JL, Cui W, Huang D, Feng YQ, et al. Study on the effect of extracts from the leaves of *Phyllanthus emblica* on immune function of mice. Zhong Yao Cai. 2013;**36**(3):441-444

[66] Kim JE, Go J, Koh EK, Song SH, Sung JE, Lee HA, Lee YH, Hong JT, Hwang DY. Gallotannin-enriched extract isolated from Galla Rhois may be a functional candidate with laxative effects for treatment of loperamide-induced constipation of SD rats. PLoS One. 2016;**11**(9):e0161144. DOI: 10.1371/journal.pone.0161144

[67] Lee SM, Lee JW, Park JD, Kim JI. Study on formation and development of *schlechtendalis chinensis* gall in *Rhus javanica*. Korean Journal of Applied Entomology. 1997;**36**:83-87

[68] Kim SH, Park HH, Lee S, Jun CD, Choi BJ, Kim SY, et al. The anti-anaphylactic effect of the gall of *Rhus javanica* is mediated through inhibition of histamine release and inflammatory cytokine secretion. International Immunopharmacology. 2005;**5**:1820-1829. DOI: 10.1016/j.intimp.2005.06.007

[69] Go J, Kim JE, Koh EK, Song SH, Seung JE, Park CK, et al. Hepatotoxicity and nephrotoxicity of gallotannin-enriched extract isolated from Galla Rhois in ICR mice. Laboratory Animal Research. 2015;**31**:101-110. DOI: 10.5625/lar.2015.31.3.101

[70] Lee JJ, Kim DH, Lim JJ, Kim DG, Min WG, Kim GS, et al. Anticoccidial effect of supplemental dietary Galla Rhois against infection with *Eimeria tenella* in chickens. Avian Pathology. 2012;**41**:403-407. DOI: 10.1080/03079457.2012.702888

[71] Cha CN, Yu EA, Park EK, Kim S, Lee HJ. Effects of dietary supplementation with Galla Rhois on growth performance and diarrhea incidence in postweaning piglets. Journal of Veterinary Clinics. 2013;**30**:353-358

[72] Ahn YJ, Lee CO, Kweon JH, Ahn JW, Park JH. Growth-inhibitory effects of derived tannins on intestinal bacteria. Journal of Applied Microbiology. 1998;**84**:439-443. DOI: 10.1046/j.1365-2672.1998.00363.x

[73] Chae HS, Kang OH, Choi JG, Oh YC, Lee YS, Brice OO, et al. Methyl gallate inhibits the production of interleukin-6

and nitric oxide via down-regulation of extracellular-signal regulated protein kinase in raw 264. 7 cells. American Journal of Chinese Medicine. 2010;**38**:973-983. DOI: 10.1142/S0192415X10008391

[74] Ata N, Oku T, Hattori M, Fujii H, Nakajima M, Saiki I. Inhibition by galloylglucose (GC6-10) of tumor invasion through extracellular matrix and gelatinase-mediated degradation of type IV collagens by metastatic tumor cells. Oncology Research. 1996;**8**:503-511

[75] Lee TY, Chang HH, Wang GJ, Chiu JH, Yang YY, Lin C. Water-soluble extract of *Salvia miltiorrhiza* ameliorates carbon tetrachloride-mediated hepatic apoptosis in rats. Journal of Pharmacy and Pharmacology. 2006;**58**:659-665. DOI: 10.1211/jpp.58.5.0011

[76] Korea Food and Drug Administration. The Korean Pharmacopeia. 11th ed. Seoul, Korea: Shinilbooks com; 2015

[77] Zhang L, Reddy N. Bioactive natural molecules and traditional herbs for life threatening diseases. Journal of Molecular Sciences. 2018;**2**(1):4. DOI: 10.155/2016/9872302

Chapter 6

The Management of Constipation: Current Status and Future Prospects

Masaki Maruyama, Kenya Kamimura, Moeno Sugita, Nao Nakajima, Yoshifumi Takahashi, Osamu Isokawa and Shuji Terai

Abstract

Chronic constipation, a common condition, can have remarkably negative effects on a patient's quality of life. Recent research has identified factors that may influence the prognosis of chronic constipation and suggests the need for adequate therapy. However, the major obstacles in this field were: (1) a small number of therapeutic options, (2) no clear diagnostic criteria, and (3) no effective method to collect information form the patients. These were due to the fact that bowel movement patterns vary widely among individuals, and also the functional constipation, including irritable bowel syndrome, is difficult to be distinguished from the chronic constipation. Recently, it has been demonstrated that the Rome IV diagnostic criteria of functional constipation and the Bristol stool form scale are useful for the objective evaluation and recording of stool. Based on these developments, and the increase of newly developed medicines the therapy for the constipation is significantly changing and therefore, if conventional therapy for chronic constipation is ineffective, switching of medicines is possible. Therefore, clinicians should update the information of these newly developed drugs available in clinics and diagnostic criteria. For this purpose, in this chapter, we have summarized the perspective on the current paradigm of treatment for chronic constipation focusing on recently introduced therapeutic drugs.

Keywords: chronic constipation, Rome IV diagnostic criteria, secretagogues, lubiprostone

1. Introduction

Many reports describe a high prevalence of constipation worldwide. For example, a survey conducted in North America by Higgins et al. reported prevalence rates of 12–19%, particularly among older populations [1]. Generally, research suggests that constipation reduces the patient's quality of life (QOL) to a level comparable with the negative effects of allergy or inflammatory bowel disease [2]. Despite these negative characteristics, however, a clear overview of chronic constipation has not yet been established.

The Rome IV diagnostic criteria, which were revised in 2016, are often used to evaluate functional constipation. However, these diagnostic criteria exclude irritable bowel syndrome (IBS), a prevalent condition (7–21%) that exists on a continuous spectrum with functional constipation. Notably, IBS and functional constipation may be associated with predominant symptoms such as abdominal pain or bloating, which are not necessarily predominant in all cases of constipation [3]. This suggests that IBS and functional constipation often overlap in real-world scenarios [4]. Furthermore, the diagnosis of chronic constipation, which often involves the appraisal of symptoms (including QOL measures), and associated therapies appear to be incomplete.

In addition to the lack of diagnostic and treatment methodology, the Japan Collaborative Cohort Study found evidence suggesting that a low bowel movement frequency increases the risks of cardiovascular disease (CVD), such as stroke and ischemic myocardial infarction, and of related mortality. The same study also found a high incidence of CVD among laxative users in Japan [5, 6]. Therefore, the effect of constipation indicates an increasingly poor prognosis. In this chapter, we review the present clinical practices targeting constipation and discuss newly introduced therapeutic drugs for constipation, such as secretagogues, which have recently yielded medical advances. With this review, we aim to prevent a perspective on the future treatment of chronic constipation.

2. Definition of constipation

Individual bowel movement patterns (including constipation) vary widely and are easily affected by many factors, including changes in the diet, living environment, mental status, and time course [7, 8]. Additionally, physicians and patients may hold different understandings of constipation. Consequently, the term "constipation" may encompass a broad spectrum of symptoms and situations. Despite these differences, constipation can be adequately defined as a status in which comfortable defecation is impossible, in accordance with many international clinical practice guidelines and review articles, as well as the Rome IV criteria [4, 9, 10].

3. Chronic constipation, including chronic functional constipation and IBS

Constipation can be roughly classified as acute or chronic, each of which can be further divided according to an organized or functional pathogenic mechanism. However, this chapter will discuss specifically chronic functional constipation in adult patients and its deleterious effects on the long-term QOL. Previously, the Rome III criteria were used to diagnose chronic functional constipation when a stringent definition is required for research purposes. In May 2016, however, the revised Rome IV criteria were published [10] (**Table 1**). Notably, these updated criteria include the requirement of other symptoms associated with difficulty of defecation and incompleteness of evacuation, as well as symptoms associated with constipation, and do not diagnose chronic functional constipation based on the frequency of bowel movements alone. Of note, these criteria require the exclusion of IBS prior to a diagnosis of chronic functional constipation (**Table 2**). However, this condition overlaps with IBS in many clinical cases. Accordingly, we recommend that in actual clinical settings, cases in which a patient's continued inability to defecate comfortably that has deleterious effects on daily life should be managed

Diagnostic criteria[a] for functional constipation (FC)
1. Must include 2 or more of the following:[b]
a. Straining during more than one-fourth (25%) of defecations
b. Lumpy or hard stools (Bristol Stool Form Scale: BSFS 1-2) more than one-fourth (25%) of defecations
c. Sensation of incomplete evacuation more than one-fourth (25%) of defecations
d. Sensation of anorectal obstruction/blockage more than one-fourth (25%) of defecations
e. Manual maneuvers to facilitate more than one fourth (25%) of defecations (e.g., digital evacuation, support of the pelvic floor)
f. Fewer than 3 spontaneous bowel movements per week
2. Loose stools are rarely present without the use of laxatives
3. Insufficient criteria for irritable bowel syndrome

[a]*Criteria fulfilled for the last 3 months with symptom onset at least 6 months prior to diagnosis.*
[b]*For research studies, patients meeting criteria for Opioid-Induced Constipation (OIC) should not be given a diagnosis of FC because it is difficult to distinguish between opioid side effects and other causes of constipation. However, clinicians recognize that these 2 conditions might overlap.*

Table 1.
The diagnostic criteria for functional constipation: This criteria is cited from "Mearin et al. [10]".

Diagnostic criteria[a] for irritable bowel syndrome
Recurrent abdominal pain, on average, at least a day per week in the last 3 months, associated with 2 or more of the following criteria:
1. Related to defecation
2. Associated with a change in frequency of stool
3. Associated with a change in form (appearance) of stool

[a]*Criteria fulfilled for the last 3 months with symptom onset at least 6 months before diagnosis.*

Table 2.
The diagnostic criteria for irritable bowel syndrome: This criteria is cited from "Mearin, et al. [10]".

as chronic constipation, even if the Rome IV criteria are not fulfilled [4]. Later, we discuss the diagnosis and management of chronic constipation, including chronic functional constipation and IBS.

3.1 Alarming symptoms associated with chronic constipation

Particular attention should be given to the management of constipation associated with alarming symptoms, which may correlate with a poor outcome due to the required therapy for an underlying disease or surgically treated condition. Patients with alarming symptoms should be further scrutinized and subjected to additional diagnostic testing before treatment is administered for constipation. Potentially alarming symptoms may include a change in stool caliber, heme-positive stool, iron-deficiency anemia, obstructive symptoms, an age of >50 years with no history of colon cancer screening, recent onset of constipation, rectal bleeding, rectal prolapse, and weight loss [9–11]. Such symptoms should be considered an indication for colonoscopy.

3.2 Secondary constipation

Secondary constipation should be excluded prior to a diagnosis of functional or chronic constipation due to IBS, as underlying high-risk diseases and etiologies must be identified [4, 10, 11]. Secondary constipation can be subdivided coarsely into drug-induced and symptomatic cases. Consequently, a diagnostic interview for chronic constipation should inquire about the time of onset, duration of disease, frequency of bowel movements, consistency of stool, symptoms associated with constipation, and the presence of concrete situations of dyschezia (e.g., abdominal pain and/or bloating, sensation of incomplete evacuation, need for manual maneuvers to facilitate defecation, and evacuation time). A clinical history, including lifestyle factors and dietary fiber and fluid intake, should also be taken. A systemic physical examination that includes a digital rectal examination (palpation for gastrointestinal mass, anorectal inspection to assess fecal impaction, stricture, rectal prolapse, rectocele, paradoxical or nonrelaxing puborectalis activity, and rectal mass), laboratory analyses (complete blood counts, biochemical profile, calcium and glucose levels, and thyroid function tests) and colonoscopy is also required to exclude secondary constipation. In summary, underlying diseases and drug-affected constipation should be considered in an evaluation of chronic constipation.

3.2.1 Underlying diseases

The diagnosis and treatment of underlying diseases is very important in the management of chronic constipation. Underlying diseases that may cause chronic constipation are listed below [9]:

Mechanical obstruction: colorectal tumor, diverticulosis, stricture, external compression from tumor/other structures, large rectocele, megacolon, postoperative abnormalities, and anal fissure.

Neurological disorders/neuropathy: autonomic neuropathy, cerebrovascular disease, cognitive impairment/dementia, depression, multiple sclerosis, Parkinson's disease, and spinal cord pathology.

Endocrine/metabolic conditions: chronic kidney disease (CKD), dehydration, diabetes mellitus, heavy metal poisoning, hypercalcemia, hypermagnesemia, hyperparathyroidism, hypokalemia, hypomagnesemia, hypothyroidism, multiple endocrine neoplasia II, and porphyria.

Gastrointestinal disorders and local painful conditions: IBS, abscess, anal fissure, fistula, hemorrhoids, levator ani syndrome, megacolon, proctalgia fugax, rectal prolapse, rectocele, and volvulus.

Myopathies: amyloidosis, dermatomyositis, scleroderma, and systemic sclerosis.

Dietary causes: dieting, fluid depletion, low fiber intake, anorexia, dementia, and depression.

Other causes: cardiac disease, degenerative joint disease, and immobility.

3.2.2 Drug-induced constipation

When evaluating a case of chronic constipation, the patient's current profile of medicine use must be understood precisely and considered during further treatment. A list of drugs that may cause chronic constipation is provided below [9].

Prescription drugs: antidepressants, antiepileptics, antihistamines, antiparkinson drugs, antipsychotics, antispasmodics, calcium channel blockers, diuretics, monoamine oxidase inhibitors, opiates, sympathomimetics, tricyclic antidepressants, and statins.

Self-medication (i.e., over-the-counter drugs): antacids (containing aluminum and calcium), antidiarrheal agents, calcium and iron supplements, and nonsteroidal anti-inflammatory drugs.

4. Diagnostic approaches to the treatment of chronic constipation

An interview based on the diagnostic criteria (**Table 1**) for functional constipation is useful when planning treatment for chronic constipation. The simple and objective Bristol stool form scale, which is used worldwide, is particularly useful for enabling an evaluation and record of the stool form and thus elucidating an individual patient's defecation status [12, 13]. When possible, the patient should maintain a stool diary that includes the number of bowel movements per day and stool consistency (Bristol stool form types 1–7, **Figure 1**) for approximately 1 week. This record is also useful for evaluating symptoms and sensations (e.g., sensation of incomplete evacuation, abdominal pain, and/or bloating) after evacuation [4].

The Bristol scale can also be used to estimate the colonic transit time. Currently, cases of functional constipation are categorized as normal-transit, slow-transit, or defecatory rectal evacuation disorder [10]. A previous histological analysis reported that slow-transit constipation results from a reduction in Cajal cells [14], suggesting that this type is caused by a decrease in the statuses of lower postprandial phasic responses (e.g., the disappearance of bowel peristalsis) [15]. Other research indicates that defecatory rectal evacuation disorders are caused by functional failures (e.g., pelvic floor line coordination disturbance) [16]. Although Bristol stool form types 1 and 2 can be attributed to slower transit constipation and types 6 and 7 are characteristic of rapid transit constipation [17], patients who meet the diagnostic criteria for functional constipation often exhibit characteristics of slow colonic transit constipation [18]. Still, the diagnosis of defecatory rectal evacuation disorders does not require diagnostic colonic and anorectal testing [19].

An improved QOL is among the most important goals of treatment for chronic constipation. Accordingly, various questionnaires are useful during the processes of diagnosis and treatment (see Section 5). If initial conservative medical management does not cure chronic constipation, additional measures such as the balloon expulsion test [8, 20, 21], manometric assessment [20], defecography [22], and radio-opaque marker testing of the whole-gut transit time should be considered [23]. Additional tests may also be performed, although the availability may be limited to certain medical centers or countries. Accordingly, interinstitutional cooperation is important.

Type 1	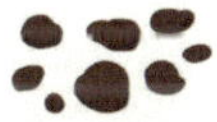	Separate hard lumps, like nuts (hard to pass)
Type 2	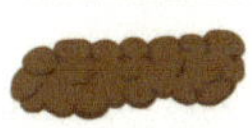	Sausage-shaped but lumpy
Type 3	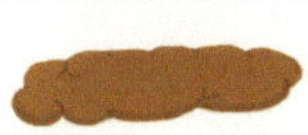	Like a sausage, but with cracks on the surface
Type 4	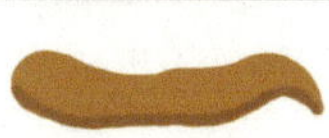	Like a sausage or snake, smooth and soft
Type 5	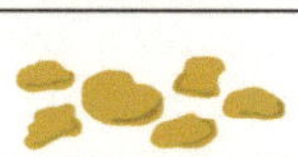	Soft blobs with clear-cut edges (passed easily)
Type 6	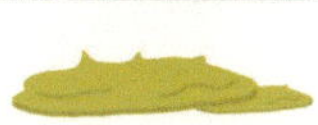	Fluffy pieces with ragged edges, a mushy stool
Type 7	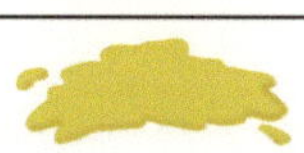	Watery, no solid pieces (entirely liquid)

Figure 1.
The Bristol Stool Form Scale: This scale is a useful tool to evaluate stool and can evaluate colonic transit time

5. Self-reported questionnaires for diagnostic purposes

Questionnaire-based self-report measures can be classified by the type of QOL evaluation and type of constipation severity quantitation. Various methods are currently advocated, although further progress in this area is needed [24]. The questionnaires most frequently mentioned in a literature search via the PubMed database are shown below.

5.1 Evaluation of severity of constipation

Constipation scoring system (CSS) [25]. The CSS comprises eight questionnaire items to assess the frequency of bowel movements, difficult or painful evacuation, completeness of evacuation, abdominal pain, time per attempt, type of assistance (including laxatives, digitation, or enemas), number of unsuccessful attempts at evacuation in a 24-h period, and duration of constipation. All but one item are scored on a 5-point Likert scale (range: 0–4); the type of assistance, including laxatives, is scored on a 3-point scale (range: 0–2). A cutoff score of 15 is used to indicate constipation.

Patient assessment of constipation symptoms (PAC-SYM) [26]. The PAC-SYM was validated for the assessment of chronic functional constipation in 216 adult patients in the USA. This tool includes 12 items to assess abdominal, rectal, and stool factors. The items are scored on a 5-point Likert scale (range: 0–4), with a score of 4 indicating the worst symptom severity. The total possible scores for the PAC-SYM range from 0 to 48, and no diagnostic cutoff score has been reported. This questionnaire has a 7-point Likert scale for four items of abdominal symptoms and three items of rectal symptoms (e.g., abdominal pain, bloating, and rectal burning) from no discomfort to very severe discomfort.

5.2 QOL evaluation tool

Gastrointestinal symptom rating scale (GSRS) [27]. The GSRS is a questionnaire comprising 15 items intended to address common gastrointestinal symptoms. The scale can be completed by the patient within approximately 5 min, and the items are scored on a 7-point Likert scale ranging from no discomfort to very severe discomfort. For evaluation purposes, a mean scale score is calculated for the equivalent of items (e.g., heart burn, nausea, and abdominal pain), and a high score indicates more severe symptoms.

Patient assessment of constipation quality of life (PAC-QOL) [28]. The PAC-QOL is a simple self-reported questionnaire used to measure the patient's QOL associated with constipation, including daily behavioral and therapeutic aspects relevant to constipation during the previous 2 week period. The PAC-QOL comprises 28 items divided into four subscales that address the patient's worries/concerns relevant to constipation, physical discomfort, psychosocial discomfort, and satisfaction. The items are scored on a 5-point scale, and a higher score indicates a lower QOL. The original edition was developed in English and has since been translated into many languages.

6. Practical treatment

In this section, we aim to provide an overview of the various available treatments for chronic constipation for which the details have been published. Patient education is a very important first step in the therapeutic management of chronic constipation [3]. Patients should be instructed to consume an adequate quantity of dietary fiber (total fiber intake: 20–30 g/day), set a routine of regular toilet time after mealtimes, and take an on-defecation position involving elevation of the lower limbs. If such measures are ineffective, an oral fiber supplement, such as psyllium (up to 30 mg/day in divided doses) may be attempted [29].

Drug therapy should be initiated if the above-described lifestyle modifications fail to treat chronic constipation, and this should be accompanied by an assessment of bowel movements every 2–4 weeks to determine the therapeutic effects. Generally, osmotic laxatives (e.g., lactulose, lactitol, mannitol, and sorbitol) are administered initially as these are cost-effective and have few adverse effects [18, 30]. Although saline laxatives (e.g., magnesium sulfate) are frequently administered in Japan, these drugs are not widely accepted worldwide and have only been evaluated clinically in small-scale randomized controlled trials (RCTs) [31]. Furthermore, patients with renal failure face the risk of serious hypermagnesemia consequent to the use of magnesium sulfate [32]. However, this drug should be considered, given its low cost and abundant use in Japan. Polyethylene glycol laxatives (17–34 g/day) should also be considered, as many RCTs have indicated that these agents are more effective than lactulose [33, 34].

If chronic constipation remains unresolved by the above therapies, newer medicines should be considered. Recent years have seen the rapid development of novel agents such as secretagogues (e.g., lubiprostone and linaclotide). However, as the availability and indications of these new drugs for chronic constipation vary among countries, all medical treatment for chronic constipation should comply with national clinical practice guidelines or guiding principle. Finally, surgical or biofeedback treatment should be considered for cases of chronic constipation that cannot be resolved with medication and patients with defecatory rectal evacuation disorders [35, 36].

7. New therapeutic drugs for chronic constipation

The extensive development of novel drugs for chronic constipation has led to variability in the potential applications among countries. For example, neither secretagogues (e.g., plecanatide) nor serotonergic enterokinetic agents (e.g., prucalopride and selective 5-hydroxytryptamine receptor agonists) have been approved for use in Japan. Below, we comment mainly on the new therapeutic drugs for chronic constipation that have been authorized for use in Japan.

7.1 Lubiprostone

Various studies have analyzed lubiprostone, the most well-developed one of the newer class of drugs. The mechanism of action of this constipation-targeting drug is interesting. Lubiprostone is a selective type-2 chloride channel (ClC-2 channel) activator. This biogenic bicyclic fatty acid was developed by Cuppoletti and Ueno for the treatment of chronic constipation and has been approved for use worldwide after the initial authorization for manufacturing and marketing in the US and Japan. [37, 38] Lubiprostone is the first clinically applied secretagogue, and accordingly, a broad range of clinical experience is associated with this drug. Moreover, the mechanism of action of this drug has been analyzed in much greater detail relative to secretagogues introduced subsequently. Specifically, this drug activates ClC-2 channels expressed in the apical membranes of intestinal epithelial cells and exerts its laxative function by inducing the secretion of intestinal fluids. The ability of lubiprostone to improve constipation symptoms has been validated through RCTs

[39], which reported the maintenance of efficacy throughout a 48-week administration period with no significant side effects [40].

Lubiprostone promotes the secretion of intestinal fluid by activating ClC-2 channels. Upon absorption from the small intestine, lubiprostone is degraded immediately to an inactive metabolite. Therefore, the effects of this drug are tissue selective, and few side effects have been observed. In the small intestine, lubiprostone activates the ClC-2 channels expressed on mucosal epithelial cells to promote the transport of chloride ions from the visceral lumen and concomitant countertransport of cations into the lumen. This activity induces a difference in the local osmotic pressure across the epithelial cell membrane, and the resulting secretion of intestinal fluid expedites defecation [41, 42]. As the expression of the ClC-2 channel is not expected to vary according to age, sex, or race, lubiprostone may be effective in elderly patients with constipation.

Clinical usefulness of lubiprostone for chronic constipation. As mentioned above, multiple RCTs have validated the effectiveness of lubiprostone for chronic constipation [39] and demonstrated a both sustained efficacy and a lack of serious adverse effects during a 48-week period of administration. The most common side effects of this drug include nausea (frequency: 19.8%), diarrhea (9.7%), abdominal distension (6.9%), headache (6.9%), and abdominal pain (5.2%) [40]. Recently, the mechanism of action of lubiprostone as a therapeutic drug for constipation was investigated in detail (see below.) Notably, a study based on a questionnaire regarding QOL, work productivity, and lifestyle impairment found that lubiprostone improved both symptoms related to chronic constipation and the patients' QOL [43]. In a phase 3 trial, Fukudo et al. found that long-term lubiprostone administration was associated with an average increase in the average spontaneous bowel movement (SBM) number per week and an improved QOL among Japanese patients with chronic idiopathic constipation [44]. In a randomized, double-blind, placebo-controlled trial of the effects of lubiprostone on chronic idiopathic constipation in diabetic patients, Christie et al. found that this drug reduced the colon transit time and increased the SBM number safely and effectively [45].

Parkinson's disease: Parkinson's disease is a very common neurodegenerative disorder characterized by motility disturbances. Constipation occurs very frequently in affected patients and is a predictor of the onset of movement disorder. Constipation appears as a symptom prior to more obvious signs of parkinsonism before disappearance of dopamine cells in substantia nigra. Accordingly, clinicians should consider the early detection of a movement disorder when evaluating cases of constipation. In a double-blind RCT of the efficacy and tolerability of lubiprostone in patients with Parkinson's disease with constipation, Ondo et al. concluded that the drug was well tolerated and effective when administered for a short duration [46].

Efficacy of lubiprostone for CKD: Mishima et al. demonstrated clearly that lubiprostone could inhibit an exacerbation of adenine-induced CKD by altering the intestinal environment or intestinal flora. That study suggested that in a patient with CKD, the intestinal tract acts as a conduit for uremic toxin excretion that is comparable with hemodialysis and urine. Lubiprostone may, therefore, be a novel therapeutic drug for CKD [47].

Protective effects on the small intestine and "leaky gut syndrome." The small intestine serves as a barrier for the selective transport of molecules in and out of the gastrointestinal tract. Failure of this barrier function renders the patient unable to absorb the nutrient for use as energy and can enable the transport of microbial pathogens and harmful chemical substances into the interior of the body. This state is known as the "leaky gut syndrome" and is thought to induce various diseases, including gastrointestinal diseases (e.g., inflammatory bowel disease), allergies, diabetes, connective tissue diseases, and liver diseases [48]. Therefore, the prevention of leaky gut syndrome would be therapeutically valuable.

No currently available therapeutic drug can improve abnormal intestinal tract permeability in humans. However, Moeser et al. revealed that lubiprostone not only promotes the secretion of intestinal fluid by activating ClC-2 channels but also protects and restores injured small intestinal mucosa [49]. The mechanism underlying the restoration of tight junctions in the mucosa remains unknown, although the ClC-2 channel was found to play an important role in restoring the tight-junction structure and barrier function in a mouse model of colitis [48]. Furthermore, Kato et al. demonstrated that lubiprostone could improve intestinal permeability in humans [50]. Although these research findings require validation, lubiprostone appears to be a promising treatment for leaky gut syndrome.

Anti-inflammatory effect. Experimentally, lubiprostone was shown to prevent indomethacin-induced intestinal disease through a mechanism dependent on the prostaglandin EP4 receptor subtype in male Sprague-Dawley rats. This effect might suppress excessive intestinal motility and promote intestinal fluid secretion, while controlling bacterial invasion and inducible nitric oxide synthase/tumor necrosis factor alpha expression, the main pathological events of intestinal disease. However, it is difficult to understand how the protective effect of lubiprostone would rely on the direct activation of the cystic fibrosis transmembrane regulator/ClC-2 channel [51].

Promotion of mucin secretion. Lubiprostone has been shown to promote mucin secretion in the small intestinal mucosa via a prostaglandin-like action and thus maintain digestive function [51]. Lubiprostone might also promote the intestinal transit of feces by providing lubrication and could thus improve the likelihood of comfortable defecation [52, 53].

Lubiprostone in clinic. A previous report indicated a correlation of Munchausen syndrome with the overuse of stimulant laxatives [54], which presents a challenge regarding dependence on these drugs. We, therefore, investigated whether lubiprostone administration would facilitate a reduction in the dose of a continuously administered stimulant laxative. In real clinics, we have shown the successful reduction or cessation of the stimulant laxative (e.g., sodium picosulfate, senna) in more than 50% of cases (n = 21) within 6 months of administering lubiprostone (manuscript in preparation). Notably, no further medications were needed in these cases. These clinical experiences suggested us that the lubiprostone may be useful not only for the symptom itself but also for the reduction of stimulant laxatives leading to the safe and cost effective treatment of constipation.

7.2 Linaclotide

Linaclotide is a newly developed therapeutic drug for chronic constipation and constipation-predominant IBS. This drug is absorbed at low levels and has few adverse effects, of which the main complaint is diarrhea [55]. This peptide drug comprises 14 amino acids and acts by binding to the guanylate cyclase C (GC-C) receptor expressed on intestinal epithelial cells, which promotes the secretion of fluids into the intestinal lumen. The GC-C receptor is associated with bodily fluid and ionic homeostasis, bowel movements, and relief from afferent pain signaling and is thus considered a therapeutic target for chronic constipation and constipation-predominant IBS [56].

When compared with placebo, linaclotide yielded excellent results in terms of the reduction in abdominal pain and increase in complete SBMs at 12 weeks after the initial first administration [57]. Furthermore, linaclotide was associated with a significant increase in the average QOL score relative to placebo in a questionnaire-based survey [58]. A cost-effectiveness analysis study revealed that the less expensive linaclotide yielded equivalent patient satisfaction to that achieved with lubiprostone [59]. As chronic constipation overlaps partially with constipation-predominant IBS, linaclotide may greatly expand the treatment options for constipation. Although linaclotide has been prescribed widely at our hospital at an appropriate once-daily dosage of 0.5 mg, we presume that many physicians may initiate this drug at a daily dosage of 0.25 mg to avoid adverse effects.

7.3 Elobixibat

Bile acids are synthesized from cholesterol in the liver and secreted to the duodenum, where they play an essential role in lipid digestion and absorption. Upon reaching the terminal ileum, bile acids are absorbed solely by the ileal bile acid transporter (IBAT) expressed only in the terminal ileum [60]. Here, 95% of the bile acids are reabsorbed through the portal system and are reconjugated and reexcreted into bile by hepatocytes in an enterohepatic cycle that occurs 2–15 times daily. Unabsorbed bile acids are transported to the colon, where they encourage the secretion of water into the large bowel lumen and thus promote large bowel movement [61, 62]. Accordingly, the administration of ursodeoxycholic acid or the occurrence of ileal diseases that enable the transport of excess amounts of bile acids to the large bowel can cause diarrhea [60].

The drug elobixibat specifically inhibits the IBAT required for bile acid reabsorption and is thus commercially available as the first IBAT inhibitor. Through its inhibitory actions, elobixibat increases the entry of bile acids into the large bowel and thus promotes evacuation. When administered orally, this drug is absorbed at low levels; accordingly, it has few adverse effects and is considered safe [63]. In Japan, elobixibat is administered orally at a once-daily dosage of 10 mg before a meal. However, the usage of this drug may vary among countries and should be confirmed carefully. To date, elobixibat has been used in only seven cases at our hospital in the short time since it has been licensed. Although only two patients have used this drug continuously for at least 2 months, all treated patients have achieved complete SBM. Elobixbat appears to act simultaneously as a stool softener and laxative stimulant. We expect that the use of this drug will increase.

7.4 Naldemedine

Naldemedine, a peripherally acting μ-opioid receptor antagonist, was developed as a therapeutic drug for opioid-induced constipation and is approved in the US and Japan [64]. This new class medication showed important therapeutic effect in improving opioid-induced constipation without reducing the efficacy of opioid drugs because it selectively targets the peripheral μ-opioid receptor as demonstrated in two-phase 3 trials [65, 66]. Therefore, although opioid-induced constipation has been initially treated with conventional laxatives, however, based on these evidences, naldemedine is expected to become a leading therapy for cases using opioids. Recently, we are switching to naldemedine to manage the constipation in cases using opioid, and approximately one-third of patients using opioids have been treated with naldemedine and showed the safe and effective bowel movement (manuscript in preparation).

8. Conclusion

To improve the QOL in the cases suffered with chronic constipation, the appropriate therapeutic intervention is essential. With the rise in the therapeutic options and its real world data, and the objective assessment methods, its treatment is dramatically changing. It is obvious that the correct diagnosis excluding the emergent situation is essential; however, the physicians need to update the information for these newly developed medicines useful for constipation and switch from the conventional agents for better QOL.

As the appropriate use of these new agents under various conditions remains uncertain, therefore, the accumulation of the clinical information, real-world data are necessary. For this purpose, this review overviewed the symptoms, diagnosis, and medicines available to date. We hope that these informations are useful for physicians treating patients and that various pathophysiological studies will elucidate the correct use of these new anticonstipation agents.

Furthermore, we hope that the development of a more ideal questionnaire will enable effective decisions regarding the most effective treatment for chronic constipation.

Conflict of interest

The authors declare that they have no current financial arrangement or affiliation with any organization that may have a direct influence on their work.

Author details

Masaki Maruyama[1], Kenya Kamimura[2*], Moeno Sugita[1], Nao Nakajima[1], Yoshifumi Takahashi[1], Osamu Isokawa[1] and Shuji Terai[2]

1 Department of Gastroenterology, Kashiwazaki General Hospital and Medical Center, Kashiwazaki, Niigata, Japan

2 Division of Gastroenterology and Hepatology, Graduate School of Medical and Dental Sciences, Niigata University, Niigata, Japan

*Address all correspondence to: kenya-k@med.niigata-u.ac.jp

References

[1] Higgins PD, Johanson JF. Epidemiology of constipation in North America: A systematic review. The American Journal of Gastroenterology. 2004;**99**:750-759. DOI: 10.1111/j.1572-0241.2004.04114.x

[2] Belsey J, Greenfield S, Candy D, Geraint M. Systematic review: Impact of constipation on quality of life in adults and children. Alimentary Pharmacology & Therapeutics. 2010;**31**:938-949. DOI: 10.1111/j.1365-2036.2010.04273.x

[3] Chey WD, Kurlander J, Eswaran S. Irritable bowel syndrome: A clinical review. Journal of the American Medical Association. 2015;**313**:949-958. DOI: 10.1001/jama.2015.0954

[4] Rao SS, Rattanakovit K, Patcharatrakul T. Diagnosis and management of chronic constipation in adults. Nature Reviews. Gastroenterology & Hepatology. 2016;**13**:295-305. DOI: 10.1038/nrgastro.2016.53

[5] Kubota Y, Iso H, Tamakoshi A. Bowel movement frequency, laxative use, and mortality from coronary heart disease and stroke among Japanese men and women: The Japan collaborative cohort (JACC) study. Journal of Epidemiology. 2016;**26**:242-248. DOI: 10.2188/jea.JE20150123

[6] Honkura K, Tomata Y, Sugiyama K, Kaiho Y, Watanabe T, Zhang S, et al. Defecation frequency and cardiovascular disease mortality in Japan: The Ohsaki cohort study. Atherosclerosis. 2016;**246**:251-256. DOI: 10.1016/j.atherosclerosis.2016.01.007

[7] Herz MJ, Kahan E, Zalevski S, Aframian R, Kuznitz D, Reichman S. Constipation: A different entity for patients and doctors. Family Practice. 1996;**13**:156-159

[8] Bharucha AE, Pemberton JH, Locke GR 3rd. American Gastroenterological Association technical review on constipation. Gastroenterology. 2013;**144**:218-238. DOI: 10.1053/j.gastro.2012.10.028

[9] Lindberg G, Hamid SS, Malfertheiner P, Thomsen OO, Fernandez LB, Garisch J, et al. World gastroenterology organisation global guideline: Constipation–a global perspective. Journal of Clinical Gastroenterology. 2011;**45**:483-487. DOI: 10.1097/MCG.0b013e31820fb914

[10] Mearin F, Lacy BE, Chang L, Chey WD, Lembo AJ, Simren M, et al. Bowel disorders. Gastroenterology. 2016. DOI: 10.1053/j.gastro.2016.02.031

[11] Wald A. Constipation: Advances in diagnosis and treatment. Journal of the American Medical Association. 2016;**315**:185-191. DOI: 10.1001/jama.2015.16994

[12] O'Donnell LJ, Virjee J, Heaton KW. Detection of pseudodiarrhoea by simple clinical assessment of intestinal transit rate. BMJ. 1990;**300**:439-440. DOI: 10.1136/bmj.300.6722.439

[13] Longstreth GF, Thompson WG, Chey WD, Houghton LA, Mearin F, Spiller RC. Functional bowel disorders. Gastroenterology. 2006;**130**:1480-1491. DOI: 10.1053/j.gastro.2005.11.061

[14] He CL, Burgart L, Wang L, Pemberton J, Young-Fadok T, Szurszewski J, et al. Decreased interstitial cell of cajal volume in patients with slow-transit constipation. Gastroenterology. 2000;**118**:14-21. DOI: 10.1016/S0016-5085(00)70409-4

[15] O'Brien MD, Camilleri M, von der Ohe MR, Phillips SF, Pemberton JH, Prather CM, et al. Motility and tone of the left colon in constipation: A role in

clinical practice? The American Journal of Gastroenterology. 1996;**91**:2532-2538

[16] Rao SS, Welcher KD, Leistikow JS. Obstructive defecation: A failure of rectoanal coordination. The American Journal of Gastroenterology. 1998;**93**:1042-1050. DOI: 10.1111/j.1572-0241.1998.00326.x

[17] Lewis SJ, Heaton KW. Stool form scale as a useful guide to intestinal transit time. Scandinavian Journal of Gastroenterology. 1997;**32**:920-924. DOI: 10.3109/00365529709011203

[18] Ford AC, Moayyedi P, Lacy BE, Lembo AJ, Saito YA, Schiller LR, et al. American College of Gastroenterology monograph on the management of irritable bowel syndrome and chronic idiopathic constipation. The American Journal of Gastroenterology. 2014;**109**(Suppl 1):S2-S26; quiz S27. DOI: 10.1038/ajg.2014.187

[19] Rao SS, Bharucha AE, Chiarioni G, Felt-Bersma R, Knowles C, Malcolm A, et al. Functional anorectal disorders. Gastroenterology. 2016. DOI: 10.1053/j.gastro.2016.02.009

[20] Bove A, Pucciani F, Bellini M, Battaglia E, Bocchini R, Altomare DF, et al. Consensus statement AIGO/SICCR: Diagnosis and treatment of chronic constipation and obstructed defecation (part I: Diagnosis). World Journal of Gastroenterology. 2012;**18**:1555-1564. DOI: 10.3748/wjg.v18.i14.1555

[21] Ratuapli S, Bharucha AE, Harvey D, Zinsmeister AR. Comparison of rectal balloon expulsion test in seated and left lateral positions. Neurogastroenterology and Motility. 2013;**25**:e813-e820. DOI: 10.1111/nmo.12208

[22] Pelsang RE, Rao SS, Welcher K. FECOM: A new artificial stool for evaluating defecation. The American Journal of Gastroenterology. 1999;**94**:183-186. DOI: 10.1111/j.1572-0241.1999.00793.x

[23] Remes-Troche JM, Rao SS. Diagnostic testing in patients with chronic constipation. Current Gastroenterology Reports. 2006;**8**:416-424

[24] McCrea GL, Miaskowski C, Stotts NA, Macera L, Hart SA, Varma MG. Review article: Self-report measures to evaluate constipation. Alimentary Pharmacology & Therapeutics. 2008;**27**:638-648. DOI: 10.1111/j.1365-2036.2008.03626

[25] Agachan F, Chen T, Pfeifer J, Reissman P, Wexner SD. A constipation scoring system to simplify evaluation and management of constipated patients. Diseases of the Colon and Rectum. 1996;**39**:681-685. DOI: 10.1007/BF02056950

[26] Frank L, Kleinman L, Farup C, Taylor L, Miner P Jr. Psychometric validation of a constipation symptom assessment questionnaire. Scandinavian Journal of Gastroenterology. 1999;**34**:870-877. DOI: 10.1080/003655299750025327

[27] Revicki DA, Wood M, Wiklund I, Crawley J. Reliability and validity of the gastrointestinal symptom rating scale in patients with gastroesophageal reflux disease. Quality of Life Research. 1998;**7**:75-83

[28] Marquis P, De La Loge C, Dubois D, McDermott A, Chassany O. Development and validation of the patient assessment of constipation quality of life questionnaire. Scandinavian Journal of Gastroenterology. 2005;**40**:540-551. DOI: 10.1080/00365520510012208

[29] Moayyedi P, Quigley EM, Lacy BE, Lembo AJ, Saito YA, Schiller LR, et al. The effect of fiber supplementation on irritable bowel syndrome: A systematic

review and meta-analysis. The American Journal of Gastroenterology. 2014;**109**:1367-1374. DOI: 10.1038/ajg.2014.195

[30] Suares NC, Ford AC. Prevalence of, and risk factors for, chronic idiopathic constipation in the community: Systematic review and meta-analysis. The American Journal of Gastroenterology. 2011;**106**:1582-1591; quiz 1581, 1592. DOI: 10.1038/ajg.2011.164

[31] Dupont C, Campagne A, Constant F. Efficacy and safety of a magnesium sulfate-rich natural mineral water for patients with functional constipation. Clinical Gastroenterology and Hepatology. 2014;**12**(8):1280-1287. DOI: 10.1016/j.cgh.2013.12.005

[32] Nyberg C, Hendel J, Nielsen OH. The safety of osmotically acting cathartics in colonic cleansing. Nature Reviews. Gastroenterology & Hepatology. 2010;7:557-564. DOI: 10.1038/nrgastro.2010.136

[33] Dipalma JA, Cleveland MV, McGowan J, Herrera JL. A randomized, multicenter, placebo-controlled trial of polyethylene glycol laxative for chronic treatment of chronic constipation. The American Journal of Gastroenterology. 2007;**102**:1436-1441. DOI: 10.1111/j.1572-0241.2007.01199.x

[34] Attar A, Lémann M, Ferguson A, Halphen M, Boutron MC, Flourié B, et al. Comparison of a low dose polyethylene glycol electrolyte solution with lactulose for treatment of chronic constipation. Gut. 1999;**44**:226-230. DOI: 10.1136/gut.44.2.226

[35] Bleijenberg G, Kuijpers HC. Treatment of the spastic pelvic floor syndrome with biofeedback. Diseases of the Colon and Rectum. 1987;**30**:108-111. DOI: 10.1007/BF02554946

[36] Rao SS, Benninga MA, Bharucha AE, Chiarioni G, Di Lorenzo C, Whitehead WE. ANMS-ESNM position paper and consensus guidelines on biofeedback therapy for anorectal disorders. Neurogastroenterology and Motility. 2015;**27**:594-609. DOI: 10.1111/nmo.12520

[37] Cuppoletti J, Malinowska DH, Tewari KP, Li QJ, Sherry AM, Patchen ML, et al. SPI-0211 activates T84 cell chloride transport and recombinant human ClC-2 chloride currents. American Journal of Physiology. Cell Physiology. 2004 Nov;**287**(5):C1173-C1183. Epub 2004 Jun 22

[38] Bao HF, Liu L, Self J, Duke BJ, Ueno R, Eaton DC. A synthetic prostone activates apical chloride channels in A6 epithelial cells. American Journal of Physiology. Gastrointestinal and Liver Physiology. 2008;**295**(2):G234-G251. DOI: 10.1152/ajpgi.00366.2007 Epub 2008 May 29

[39] Ford AC, Suares NC. Effect of laxatives and pharmacological therapies in chronic idiopathic constipation: Systematic review and meta-analysis. Gut. 2011;**60**:209-218. DOI: 10.1136/gut.2010.227132

[40] Lembo AJ, Johanson JF, Parkman HP, Rao SS, Miner PB Jr, Ueno R. Long-term safety and effectiveness of lubiprostone, a chloride channel (ClC-2) activator, in patients with chronic idiopathic constipation. Digestive Diseases and Sciences. 2011;**56**:2639-2645. DOI: 10.1007/s10620-011-1801-0

[41] Cuppoletti J, Malinowska DH, Tewari KP, Li QJ, Sherry AM, Patchen ML, et al. SPI-0211 activates T84 cell chloride transport and recombinant human ClC-2 chloride currents. American Journal of Physiology. Cell Physiology. 2004;**287**:C1173-C1183

[42] Bao HF, Liu L, Self J, Duke BJ, Ueno R, Eaton DC. A synthetic prostone activates apical chloride channels in A6

epithelial cells. American Journal of Physiology. Gastrointestinal and Liver Physiology. 2008;**295**:G234-G251. DOI: 10.1152/ajpgi.00366.2007

[43] Abe T, Hachiro Y, Ebisawa Y, Hishiyama H, Murakami M, Kunimoto M. Efficacy of lubiprostone in chronic constipation: Clinical and work productivity outcomes. Journal of Gastrointestinal and Digestive System. 2014;**4**:5. DOI: 10.4172/2161-069X.1000223

[44] Fukudo S, Hongo M, Kaneko H, Takano M, Ueno R. Lubiprostone increases spontaneous bowel movement frequency and quality of life in patients with chronic idiopathic constipation. Clinical Gastroenterology and Hepatology. 2015;**13**:294-301.e5. DOI: 10.1016/j.cgh.2014.08.026

[45] Christie J, Shroff S, Shahnavaz N, Carter LA, Harrison MS, Dietz-Lindo KA, et al. A randomized, double-blind, placebo-controlled trial to examine the effectiveness of lubiprostone on constipation symptoms and colon transit time in diabetic patients. The American Journal of Gastroenterology. 2017;**112**: 356-364. DOI: 10.1038/ajg.2016.531

[46] Ondo WG, Kenney C, Sullivan K, Davidson A, Hunter C, Jahan I, et al. Placebo-controlled trial of lubiprostone for constipation associated with Parkinson disease. Neurology. 2012;**78**:1650-1654. DOI: 10.1212/WNL.0b013e3182574f28

[47] Mishima E, Fukuda S, Shima H, Hirayama A, Akiyama Y, Takeuchi Y, et al. Alternation of the intestinal environment by Lubiprostone is associated with amelioration of adenine-induced CKD. Journal of the American Society of Nephrology. 2015;**26**: 1787-1794. DOI: 10.1681/ASN.2014060530

[48] Jin Y, Pridgen TA, Blikslager AT. Pharmaceutical activation or genetic absence of ClC-2 alters tight junctions during experimental colitis. Inflammatory Bowel Diseases. 2015;**21**:2747-2757. DOI: 10.1097/MIB.0000000000000550

[49] Moeser AJ, Nighot PK, Engelke KJ, Ueno R, Blikslager AT. Recovery of mucosal barrier function in ischemic porcine ileum and colon is stimulated by a novel agonist of the ClC-2 chloride channel, lubiprostone. American Journal of Physiology. Gastrointestinal and Liver Physiology. 2007;**292**:G647-G656. DOI: 10.1152/ajpgi.00183.2006

[50] Kato T, Honda Y, Kurita Y, Iwasaki A, Sato T, Kessoku T, et al. Lubiprostone improves intestinal permeability in humans, a novel therapy for the leaky gut: A prospective randomized pilot study in healthy volunteers. PLoS One. 2017;**12**:e0175626. DOI: 10.1371/journal.pone.0175626

[51] Hayashi S, Kurata N, Yamaguchi A, Amagase K, Takeuchi K. Lubiprostone prevents nonsteroidal anti-inflammatory drug-induced small intestinal damage by suppressing the expression of inflammatory mediators via EP4 receptors. The Journal of Pharmacology and Experimental Therapeutics. 2014;**349**:470-479. DOI: 10.1124/jpet.114.213991

[52] Majewski M, Sarosiek I, Wallner G, Edlavitch SA, Sarosiek J. Stimulation of mucin, mucus, and viscosity during lubiprostone in patients with chronic constipation may potentially lead to increase of lubrication. Clinical and Translational Gastroenterology. 2014;**5**:e66. DOI: 10.1038/ctg.2014.19

[53] De Lisle RC. Lubiprostone stimulates small intestinal mucin release. BMC Gastroenterology. 2012;**12**:156. DOI: 10.1186/1471-230X-12-156

[54] Oster JR, Materson BJ, Rogers AI. Laxative abuse syndrome. The American Journal of Gastroenterology. 1980;**74**:451-458

[55] Andresen V, Camilleri M. Linaclotide acetate. Drugs of the Future. 2008;**33**:570-576. DOI: 10.1358/dof.2008.033.07.1214164

[56] Góngora-Benítez M, Tulla-Puche J, Albericio F. Constella™(EU)-Linzess™(USA): The last milestone in the long journey of the peptide linaclotide and its implications for the future of peptide drugs. Future Medicinal Chemistry. 2013;**5**:291-300. DOI: 10.4155/fmc.13.5

[57] Sood R, Ford AC. Linaclotide: New mechanisms and new promise for treatment in constipation and irritable bowel syndrome. Therapeutic Advances in Chronic Disease. 2013;**4**:268-276. DOI: 10.1177/2040622313500110

[58] O'Dell KM, Rummel AE, Fang NC, Nguyen NN. Linaclotide: A guanylate cyclase type-C agonist for the treatment of constipation-predominant irritable bowel syndrome and chronic constipation. Formulary. 2012;**47**:15-22. DOI: 10.4103/0972-4958.121571

[59] Huang H, Taylor DC, Carson RT, Sarocco P, Friedman M, Munsell M, et al. Economic evaluation of linaclotide for the treatment of adult patients with chronic idiopathic constipation in the United States. Managed Care. 2016;**25**:41-48. DOI: 10.3111/13696998.2014.979291

[60] Jiang C, Xu Q, Wen X, Sun H. Current developments in pharmacological therapeutics for chronic constipation. Acta Pharmaceutica Sinica B. 2015;**5**:300-309. DOI: 10.1016/j.apsb.2015.05.006

[61] Mekjian HS, Phillips SF, Hofmann AF. Colonic secretion of water and electrolytes induced by bile acids: Perfusion studies in man. The Journal of Clinical Investigation. 1971;**50**:1569-1577. DOI: 10.1172/JCI106644

[62] Bampton PA, Dinning PG, Kennedy ML, Lubowski DZ, Cook IJ. The proximal colonic motor response to rectal mechanical and chemical stimulation. American Journal of Physiology. Gastrointestinal and Liver Physiology. 2002;**282**:G443-G449. DOI: 10.1152/ajpgi.00194.2001

[63] Acosta A, Camilleri M. Elobixibat and its potential role in chronic idiopathic constipation. Therapeutic Advances in Gastroenterology. 2014;**7**:167-175. DOI: 10.1177/1756283X14528269

[64] Markham A. Naldemedine: First global approval. Drugs. 2017;**77**:923-927. DOI: 10.1007/s40265-017-0750-0

[65] Hale M, Wild J, Reddy J, Yamada T, Arjona Ferreira JC. Naldemedine versus placebo for opioid-induced constipation (COMPOSE-1 and COMPOSE-2): Two multicentre, phase 3, double-blind, randomised, parallel-group trials. The Lancet Gastroenterology & Hepatology. 2017;**2**:555-564. DOI: 10.1016/S2468-1253(17)30105-X

[66] Katakami N, Harada T, Murata T, Shinozaki K, Tsutsumi M, Yokota T, et al. Randomized phase III and extension studies of naldemedine in patients with opioid-induced constipation and cancer. Journal of Clinical Oncology. 2017;**35**:3859-3866. DOI: 10.1200/JCO.2017.73.0853